PO
OF
Self-Care

TRANSFORMING HEART HEALTH
WITH LIFESTYLE MEDICINE

DR SUNIL KUMAR

MBBS MRCA FCAI FRSA Dip IBLM Dip BSLM
Board Certified Lifestyle Medicine Physician
and a Health Coach

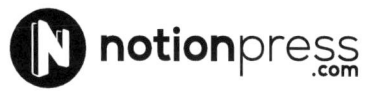

notionpress.com

INDIA · SINGAPORE · MALAYSIA

Copyright © Dr Sunil Kumar 2023
All Rights Reserved.

ISBN

Hardcase 979-8-89186-784-0
Paperback 979-8-89186-591-4

This book has been published with all efforts taken to make the material error-free after the consent of the author. However, the author and the publisher do not assume and hereby disclaim any liability to any party for any loss, damage, or disruption caused by errors or omissions, whether such errors or omissions result from negligence, accident, or any other cause.

While every effort has been made to avoid any mistake or omission, this publication is being sold on the condition and understanding that neither the author nor the publishers or printers would be liable in any manner to any person by reason of any mistake or omission in this publication or for any action taken or omitted to be taken or advice rendered or accepted on the basis of this work. For any defect in printing or binding the publishers will be liable only to replace the defective copy by another copy of this work then available.

As I take a moment to look back on the creation of this book, I am filled with a profound sense of thanks for the multitude of kindred spirits who have accompanied me on this path. To my beloved family and treasured friends, your constant belief and solid support have been the guiding light through my journey..

Equally deserving of my deepest appreciation are all my coachees. Your commitment to embracing the principles laid out in these pages and your subsequent transformations are the true testimonies of its potential. Witnessing your journeys, your challenges, and your triumphs has been a source of continuous inspiration. Every story of revitalized health and rejuvenated spirit only reinforced my belief in the importance of this work.

This book is not just an amalgamation of words and ideas, but a tapestry woven with the threads of dedication, friendship, and transformative journeys. To each one of you who has been a part of this odyssey, whether by standing by my side or by embarking on your own path to better health, thank you. You are the heartbeat of this book.

As the author of this text, I must illuminate the intent behind the repetition of themes within this book . This is not a mere exercise in literary excess; rather, it is a conscious strategy to transform reading into action. The ideas are reiterated, not to fill space, but to forge them into tools for change, to transition from passive absorption to dynamic application. My aspiration extends beyond presenting information; it is to provide a guide that prompts decisive action. Each restated concept is a steppingstone designed to facilitate the reader's journey from contemplation to execution. In this way, the book is not just a source of information but a catalyst for transformation, encouraging the reader to apply its principles proactively in the tapestry of their own lives.

Dr Sunil Kumar

Table of Contents

Foreword 7
Nurturing Myself to Nurture Others 19
Purpose of this book 23
Disclaimer 25

01 Introduction to Self-Care
    and Lifestyle Medicine.. 27
02 The Impact of Lifestyle on Heart Health............ 33
03 Self-Care Practices for a Healthy Heart 41
04 Implementing Lifestyle Medicine
    Principles for Heart Health.................................. 83
05 Monitoring and Evaluating Heart
    Health Progress... 91
06 Maintaining Long-Term Heart Health
    with Self-Care 99
07 The Power of Self-Care: Real-Life Stories
    and Inspirational Examples 109
08 Embracing Healthy Behavior Change 115
09 Conclusion: Embracing Self-Care for
    Heart Health Transformation............................ 119

Table of Contents

Resources for Further Exploration and Support......... *125*
References *127*
Self-Care Plan for Heart Health *131*
Physical Activity Prescription *135*
Heart-Healthy Recipes *137*
10 Week Self-Care Plan Incorporating
Core Principles Learnt from this Book *141*
About the Author *145*

Foreword

The Power of Self-Care: Transforming Heart Health with Lifestyle Medicine" by Dr. Sunil Kumar is not just a title but a testament to the content's depth and relatability. It resonates deeply, aptly summarizing the essence of the book. Dr. Kumar masterfully crafts a narrative tailored for its audience. It's simple enough for the everyday reader to grasp yet doesn't compromise the scientific rigor the subject demands. Each chapter in this masterpiece is a study in balance - concise enough to maintain reader interest, yet thorough enough to convey all vital details. The reader is kept engaged throughout, benefiting from a wealth of knowledge without feeling overwhelmed. Dr. Kumar's book is an invaluable resource for all - from laypersons to healthcare professionals. Given that many healthcare workers still have limited exposure to LM, "The Power of Self-Care" fills a crucial gap, offering insights and guidance on the topic. In conclusion, a hearty congratulations to Dr. Sunil Kumar for this enlightening contribution to the realm of Lifestyle Medicine. His book stands as a beacon, guiding many towards better understanding and proactive action in the domain of heart health. Wishing Dr. Kumar all the continued success he so richly deserves!

Dr Ifeoma Monye
President of the World Lifestyle Medicine Organisation WLMO,
Chairman and Founder of the Society of Lifestyle Medicine of Nigeria
President and Co-Founder of the African Lifestyle Medicine Council
Board Certified Lifestyle Medicine Physician
Fellow of the American College of Lifestyle Medicine,
Fellow of the British Society of Lifestyle Medicine
Fellow of the Royal College of General Practitioners and Sessional NHS GP
Chief Consultant Family Physician and Founder of the Brookfield Centre for Lifestyle Medicine, Abuja, Nigeria.

Foreword

It is widely acknowledged that the conventional healthcare model is unsustainable. There is a compelling need for a shift from a focus on treating ailments to emphasizing prevention, from clinician-driven approaches to empowering individuals to take control of their health. The time has come to unlock the untapped potential of self-care, which can transform individual, community, population, and healthcare system outcomes. There couldn't be a better moment to delve into this book and explore the invaluable insights it offers into sustainable solutions for healthy living and the revitalization of healthcare systems worldwide. Research and experience have underscored the risk that, if not carefully managed, 21st-century lifestyles could lead to shorter lives and more time spent battling illness and disease. Advances in food manufacturing have made unhealthy, cheap, and heavily advertised foods more accessible.

The proliferation of computers, the entertainment options provided by television and streaming services, and sedentary travel arrangements have resulted in less physically active populations. Add to this the time people spend in sedentary jobs, and we have a recipe for excessive weight gain. While there is a decline in the popularity of smoking, efforts are still needed to extinguish this practice completely and relegate it to history. Regrettably, the same cannot be said for alcohol use, which continues to expose people to its harmful effects.

The complex interplay of these developments has sadly led to an increase in lifestyle-related conditions arising from a combination of poor diets, sedentary lifestyles, substance misuse, and high-stress living. Addressing these factors and empowering more people to take charge of their health and well-being necessitates a paradigm shift that centers on access to information and knowledge, replacing the over-reliance on medications, clinics, and hospitals. It has been evident for some time that a healthcare model centered around disease treatment is unsustainable and will not lead to healthier populations. Conservative estimates suggest that healthcare plays a role in population health outcomes of no more than 20%. Therefore, it is imperative to make information and knowledge about lifestyles more readily accessible, in a simplified, user-friendly, and relatable format.

In this book, Dr. Kumar adeptly combines scientific, clinical, lifestyle medicine, and population health expertise in a format that is easy to read, understand, and put into practice. Its beauty lies in its ability to present complex information in an easily understandable manner for all audiences. For scientists and clinician-researchers, they will find evidence-based principles, concepts, approaches, and interventions. At the same time, patients and healthy individuals will appreciate the simple, straightforward guidance and advice. Dr. Kumar deserves commendation for writing something that maintains scientific rigor while being simple and relatable in its delivery.In a world inundated with various products, wellness programs, quick fixes, and miracle cures, the greatest need is for simple, evidence-based, and robust guidance that people can trust.

This book fulfills all these aspects of lifestyle medicine. It simplifies complex principles for readers, revealing the true path to lasting health through the transformative power of self-care and lifestyle medicine. While the focus is on heart health, the principles, and benefits from following the advice will positively impact the entire body and its different systems. Whether you are a clinician seeking to enhance your knowledge of lifestyle medicine or an individual searching for information to lead a healthier life, this book provides a treasure trove of knowledge, backed by the latest research and scientific principles, presented in a simple and practical manner that takes into account the challenges of 21st-century lifestyles. I trust that you will find the guidance and insights within this book to be practical and applicable—insights on how what you eat, how you move, how you manage stress, and the quality of your sleep can be the wellspring of wellness and good health. The advice offered in this book will not only add years to your life but life to your years. Enjoy!

Prof Edward Kunonga
FFPH MBA (merit) DLSHTM MSc (Lon) IBLM BSc Hons MCSP
Director of Transformation and Population Health Management NECS and NENC ICB Public Health Consultant
Lifestyle Medicine Specialist and Trustee BSLM
Visiting Professor Teesside University
Honorary Lecturer Queen Mary University London
Regional CPD Coordinator FPH Executive Advisor Zimbabwe College of Public Health Physicians

Foreword

Dr. Kumar, through his insightful book, has encapsulated his fervour and dedication towards lifestyle medicine, a field that emphasizes the importance of daily habits in fostering good health. In a world reeling and recuperating from the clutches of a pandemic, his timely narrative acts as a beacon of guidance for individuals to Armor themselves against future health adversities. This compact guide doesn't just stop at preaching the 'whys' of a healthy lifestyle, but delves into the 'how's,' equipping readers with pragmatic steps to turn the tide in their favor. The essence of his message is not just about transient changes, but a call for enduring transformation aimed at cultivating a better self. In a landscape where health has become a focal discussion, Dr. Kumar's book emerges as an essential read. It beckons to those who are on a quest not merely to survive, but to thrive by embracing a lifestyle that is in harmony with the body's natural rhythm. By igniting a discourse on proactive health measures, Dr. Kumar is not just contributing to individual wellness, but is sowing seeds of change that have the potential to ripple through communities, fostering a culture of health-conscious individuals. This book isn't just a read, but a journey towards self-realization and empowerment in taking charge of one's health, a steppingstone for anyone yearning to unveil a healthier, and thereby, a better version of themselves.

Dr Rupesh Jha
General Practitioner FRCGP Dip BSLM PGCME
Board Certified Lifestyle Physician UK

Foreword

Dr. Kumar, a highly experienced Board-Certified Lifestyle Medicine Physician and Health Coach who knows all the intricacies and intricate details of the human body blends science beautifully with self-empowerment in this book. First, I extend my heartiest congratulations to Dr Kumar on writing this book which is an absolute treasure.

Self-care is a necessity and one that is so intertwined in our physical, mental and emotional wellbeing. Caring for ourselves makes us healthier in all fronts and thus paves the way to

caring for others better. Our role and responsibility in life is to influence the modifiable factors that we are born with to better our health and in this book, we concentrate on the Cardiovascular health. Our genes and our family history come with us.

A powerful journey with promising results is what one gains through the contents of this book.

I have had the pleasure and privilege of being part of Dr Kumar's group which took us through the 10-week programme which is detailed in the book and the commitment, advice, and encouragement that he showed us has been outstanding and one that I have hardly seen anywhere. He instilled the habits deep in us and we have reaped huge benefits. This is only due to his intense commitment to enhance the wellbeing of others around him with no return other than the mental satisfaction of helping humanity and mankind.

It is well worth one's time to go through the facts in this book which are very methodically enlisted to reduce and hopefully reverse the risks in our health that each of us are accumulating. The little steps each day will lead to giant leaps in our health.

Heart disease has become increasingly common. The chapters make for very easy reading, set in simple language and one that is easy to implement on a day-to-day basis despite the busy lives that many of us lead. It is the consistency and daily habits that make the difference. The bite size lay out lends to easy understanding, implementing, and practicing.

Each chapter builds from one to the other on improving Cardiovascular health through self-care and Lifestyle Medicine in which a huge expertise of Dr Kumar lies. The practices and implementation, monitoring and evaluating progress and then maintaining it for long term is thus one layer added to the previous one. The real-life including his own stories and inspirational examples are the icing on the cake as one can always relate to a story and take it away with us.

Tips to developing healthy habits for life, strategies for motivation and consistency is very useful as one needs to implement and maintain the habits learned. The self-care takes us through elements of nutrition, physical activity, stress management, importance of sleep and social connections which form the main pillars of our wellbeing.

The heart healthy diet incorporates the importance of all components of a healthy diet and the macronutrients and role of superfoods. The physical activity enumerating effects on health, the types of exercise and developing a personalised exercise plan forms the next component. Sleep helps with heart health and establishing healthy sleep patterns and combating sleep disorders form the next prescription. Stress management section involves the effect of stress on heart health and the various ways of combating stress. Relaxation and mindfulness techniques offer benefits like no other and is a must in this fast-paced world. Social connections are also stressed to make one aware that it is an integral part of our well-being. This is thus a wholesome product.

Lifestyle medicine applications to heart health, setting realistic goals, overcoming barriers, and building a supportive network interlaces with the previous aspects. The invaluable references, recipes, plans and tips at the end are brilliant. A book written by one who has practiced it through and through always works wonders as he knows the very core of each concept that he is explaining. Resources for further support and references that are plenty in this book shows the commitment, discipline, and hard work by the author in taking all the help in here to the next level for the motivated individual and developing the inner interest that one is doing this for oneself and for the ones they care about.

The 10-week self-care plan as I have already noted is one of the most effective ones that will reap us a ton of rewards for the longer term. The final self-care plan and physical activity prescription brings in a nutshell all elements and is concise and easy to do and not a chore.

I wish Dr Sunil Kumar the very best with this book and hope to see many similar practical books which will be a massive help for the well-being of the individual and the community at large.

Dr Devika Maheswari
MBBS, MRCOG,MRCGP,FRCOG
Senior Partner at Caldergreen Medical Practice
Andrew Street
East Kilbride Lanarkshire

Foreword

This elegant and very useful book by Dr Sunil Kumar brings his medical and lifestyle knowledge and expertise together in a clear accessible manner. It gives hope to many people that they can do something about their heart health and bring about change in small manageable ways.

The advice is practical, well researched and easy to follow. Dr Kumar's compassion and passion for helping others comes through very clearly. I have personally followed the advice here and benefitted from the simple but powerful lifestyle changes described in the book.

I am recommending this book to friends and colleagues. Thank you Dr Kumar.

Dr Ananta Dave
MBBS, MD, FRCPsych, MMedEth
Chief Medical Officer
Black Country ICB NHS
Consultant Psychiatrist

Nurturing Myself to Nurture Others

My Tale of Personal and Professional Transformation

I am Dr. Sunil Kumar, a busy doctor who once found himself lost in the demanding whirlwind of the medical profession. My days were long, filled with endless work, and little time for anything else. The unhealthy routine of grab-and-go meals, no exercise, constant stress, and barely enough sleep led to a significant weight gain, affecting both my physical and mental health.

One morning, the reflection staring back at me was a wake-up call. I realized that despite being a caregiver to many, I had neglected my own well-being. It was time for a change. Drawing from my medical knowledge, I started to design a plan to restore my health through self-care principles.

I began with changing how I ate, focusing on balanced, heart-healthy meals. I made time for simple exercises like brisk walks and stretching, even during busy days at the hospital. To manage stress, I started practicing breathing exercises, writing down things I was grateful for, and spending time in nature. And to improve my sleep, I created a calm bedtime routine to help me unwind.

Though juggling self-care with hospital duties was tough, the results were worth it. By making these small yet consistent changes, I lost 25 kgs and improved my heart health significantly. I felt a new surge of energy, less pain, and a sense of calm even in the face of daily hospital chaos.

This personal transformation ignited a passion to learn more. I pursued certifications in Lifestyle Medicine from reputable institutions in the USA and the UK, and also became a certified health coach. With this new knowledge, I began helping others around me, sharing the self-care principles that had helped me. It was immensely fulfilling to see colleagues and friends transform their health too. Each success story, like a colleague losing weight or a nurse reversing her prediabetes, reinforced the powerful impact of small, sustainable lifestyle changes.

Now, through my book "The Power of Self-Care," I wish to share my journey and the valuable lessons learned. It's not just about my story, but a guide to inspire and help others prioritize their health, no matter how busy life gets. The book emphasizes that with the right steps, anyone can take control of their well-being, prevent, and manage chronic diseases, and significantly improve their quality of life. Through simple yet professional guidance, I aim to make the path of self-care accessible to all, demonstrating that even amidst the hectic pace of modern life, taking care of oneself is not just possible, but profoundly rewarding.

Purpose of this book

"The Power of Self-Care: Transforming Heart Health with Lifestyle Medicine"

Heart disease continues to be one of the leading causes of death worldwide, affecting millions each year. While genetics and family history play a role, our daily lifestyle choices have a profound impact on heart health. The good news is that we have more control over our health than we realize. By adopting simple yet effective lifestyle changes, we can significantly reduce the risk of heart disease and even reverse existing damage to the heart. In this groundbreaking book, distinguished lifestyle medicine physician

Dr. Sunil Kumar provides a holistic approach to transforming heart health through the power of self-care. Blending his extensive medical expertise with his passion for promoting wellbeing, Dr. Kumar will guide you through incorporating positive lifestyle habits to take charge of your cardiovascular wellness. This book explores the pillars of lifestyle medicine – nutrition, physical activity, stress management, sleep, and social connections – and how optimizing these key areas can

Purpose of this book

help you maintain a healthy heart. You will discover heart-healthy recipes, customizable exercise plans, stress-busting techniques, sleep hygiene strategies, and more to empower you to make sustainable changes. Transforming the health of your heart doesn't happen overnight. It requires commitment to developing healthy habits and embracing self-care as a lifelong practice. With patience and consistency, the small steps you take each day will lead to significant improvements over time. Lifestyle medicine offers a natural alternative to solely treating disease once it occurs.

By following the practical advice outlined in this book, you can begin your journey towards preventing heart disease and experiencing renewed energy and vitality. The power lies within you to take control of your heart health destiny. Are you ready to get started? Turn the page and begin learning proven techniques based in evidence-based medicine to transform your heart, health, and life for the better. The rest of your journey starts here.

Disclaimer

The information provided in this book is intended for general educational and informational purposes only. It is not intended as medical advice nor to replace professional medical care. While care has been taken to ensure that information presented is accurate and in accordance with accepted standards at the time of publication, medical information is constantly changing. Therefore, readers are urged to consult a qualified healthcare professional for advice regarding any medical condition or treatment plan.

The author and publisher expressly disclaim responsibility, loss, injury or other damages incurred from any application or use of the information provided herein. This book shares the author's personal experiences, insights, and suggestions around adopting lifestyle medicine techniques for self-care. However, each individual's health status, needs, and journey are unique. You are encouraged to adapt and apply the principles in this book based on your own needs, limitations, and under the guidance of your trusted healthcare providers.

Disclaimer

Work closely with your medical team to evaluate how applying lifestyle medicine principles can fit into your overall wellness plan in a safe, appropriate manner. The nutrition, exercise, stress management, sleep and other self-care practices discussed in this book should not be used to diagnose, treat, cure, or prevent any disease or replace medical treatment. Consult with your healthcare providers prior to changing your dietary intake, physical activity levels, sleep habits, medications or medical treatments to avoid potential adverse impacts of lifestyle changes on health status. The author has made reasonable efforts to provide current and accurate information.

However, the author makes no representations or warranties of any kind, express or implied, about the completeness or accuracy of the contents of this book. The author shall not be liable for any loss, injury, or damages incurred as a result of reliance on the contents. Your use of any information provided in this book is solely at your own risk.

Introduction to Self-Care and Lifestyle Medicine

Understanding Self-Care and its Importance

In today's fast-paced world, it is all too easy to neglect our own well-being in the pursuit of success and happiness. However, it is crucial to understand that self-care is not a luxury but a necessity, especially when it comes to maintaining a healthy heart. In this subchapter, we will delve into the concept of self-care and its significance in promoting heart health using the principles of lifestyle medicine.

Self-care encompasses a wide range of activities and practices that enhance our physical, mental, and emotional well-being. It involves taking responsibility for our own health and making conscious choices to prioritize self-care in our daily lives. While some may view self-care as indulgent or selfish, it is important to recognize that caring for ourselves is the foundation for caring for others and achieving overall well- being.

When it comes to heart health, self-care becomes even more critical. Lifestyle medicine principles emphasize the power of lifestyle choices in preventing and managing chronic diseases, including heart disease. By implementing self-care practices, we can significantly reduce the risk of developing heart-related issues and promote a healthier cardiovascular system.

Self-care for heart health involves adopting healthy eating habits, engaging in regular physical activity, managing stress effectively, getting enough sleep, and maintaining a positive mindset. These practices work synergistically to support heart health and overall well-being. For instance, a balanced diet rich in fruits, vegetables, whole grains, and lean proteins not only nourishes the body but also helps maintain healthy cholesterol levels and blood pressure.

Regular physical activity, such as walking, jogging, or cycling, strengthens the heart and improves circulation, reducing the risk of heart disease. Additionally, managing stress through techniques like meditation, deep breathing exercises, or engaging in hobbies can have a profound impact on heart health by lowering blood pressure and reducing inflammation.

Sleep, often overlooked in our busy lives, plays a vital role in heart health as well. Sufficient sleep allows the heart to rest and recover, supporting cardiovascular function and reducing the risk of heart disease. Finally, maintaining a positive mindset and engaging in activities that bring joy and fulfillment can contribute to reduced stress levels and improved heart health.

In conclusion, self-care is a powerful tool in promoting heart health using lifestyle medicine principles. By understanding the importance of self-care and implementing practices that prioritize our well-being, we can transform our heart health and lead a more fulfilling and balanced life. Remember, self-care is not selfish; it is a vital investment in our own health and happiness, ultimately enabling us to better care for others and make a positive impact on the world around us.

Defining Lifestyle Medicine and its Role in Heart Health

In today's fast-paced and stressful world, taking care of our health has become more important than ever. When it comes to heart health, adopting a lifestyle medicine approach can be a game-changer. Lifestyle medicine focuses on incorporating healthy habits into our daily lives to prevent and manage chronic diseases, including heart disease. In this subchapter, we will explore what lifestyle medicine is and how it can benefit anyone looking to improve their heart health.

Lifestyle medicine is a branch of medicine that emphasizes the use of evidence-based lifestyle interventions to prevent, treat, and even reverse chronic diseases. It recognizes that our daily choices, such as diet, physical activity, stress management, sleep, and social connections, play a significant role in our overall health, including heart health. By making positive changes in these areas, we can reduce the risk of heart disease and improve our cardiovascular well-being.

When it comes to self-care for heart health using lifestyle medicine principles, it starts with nutrition. A heart-healthy diet focuses on consuming whole, plant-based foods, such as fruits, vegetables, whole grains, legumes, and nuts. It also encourages reducing processed foods, added sugars, and unhealthy fats.

A well-balanced diet can lower cholesterol levels, manage blood pressure, and promote weight loss, all of which are crucial for a healthy heart.

Physical activity is another key component of lifestyle medicine for heart health. Engaging in regular exercise not only helps maintain a healthy weight but also strengthens the heart muscle, improves blood circulation, and reduces the risk of developing heart disease. Finding enjoyable activities and incorporating them into our daily routines can make a significant difference in our heart health journey.

Stress management is often overlooked, but it plays a vital role in heart health. Chronic stress can lead to high blood pressure, increased heart rate, and inflammation, all of which contribute to heart disease. Practicing relaxation techniques, such as deep breathing exercises, meditation, and yoga, can help reduce stress and improve cardiovascular health.

Quality sleep is essential for overall well-being, including heart health. Poor sleep has been linked to an increased risk of heart disease, high blood pressure, and obesity. Creating a sleep routine that includes a consistent bedtime, a comfortable sleep environment, and limiting screen time before bed can greatly enhance the quality of our sleep and protect our hearts.

Finally, social connections are crucial for heart health. Building and maintaining strong relationships with family, friends, and community can provide emotional support, reduce stress, and promote healthy behaviors. Engaging in social activities and staying connected with loved ones can greatly impact our heart health and overall well-being.

By understanding the principles of lifestyle medicine and incorporating them into our lives, we can take control of our heart health and transform our lives. Whether you are looking to prevent heart disease or manage existing conditions, lifestyle medicine offers a holistic approach that empowers you to make positive changes. It's never too late to start on the path to better heart health through self-care and lifestyle medicine.

The Impact of Lifestyle on Heart Health

The connection between lifestyle choices and heart disease

Your heart is a vital organ that plays a crucial role in keeping you alive and well. However, in today's fast-paced and stress-filled world, heart disease has become alarmingly common. The good news is that many cases of heart disease can be prevented or managed through lifestyle choices.

In this subchapter, we will explore the powerful connection between lifestyle choices and heart disease. By understanding this link, you will be equipped with the knowledge to transform your heart health using the principles of lifestyle medicine.

First and foremost, it is important to recognize that our choices have a profound impact on our heart health. Unhealthy habits such as smoking, excessive alcohol consumption, and a sedentary lifestyle can significantly increase your risk of developing heart disease. These habits not only damage your heart directly but also contribute to other risk factors such as high blood pressure, high cholesterol, and obesity.

On the other hand, adopting a heart-healthy lifestyle can greatly reduce your risk of heart disease and improve your overall well-being. Regular physical activity, such as brisk walking, cycling, or swimming, helps strengthen your heart and cardiovascular system. Additionally, it promotes weight management, reduces stress, and improves mood.

Eating a balanced diet rich in fruits, vegetables, whole grains, lean proteins, and healthy fats is another crucial aspect of maintaining heart health. By avoiding processed foods, excessive salt, and saturated fats, you can lower your cholesterol levels and blood pressure, reducing the strain on your heart.

Managing stress is also essential in preventing heart disease. Chronic stress can lead to high blood pressure, inflammation, and unhealthy coping mechanisms such as overeating or excessive drinking. Adopting stress-reduction techniques such as meditation, deep breathing exercises, or engaging in hobbies can significantly improve your heart health.

Furthermore, adequate sleep is crucial for heart health. Poor sleep quality or insufficient sleep can increase the risk of high blood pressure, obesity, and diabetes –

all of which contribute to heart disease. Establishing a relaxing bedtime routine, ensuring a comfortable sleep environment, and prioritizing sleep are key in maintaining a healthy heart.

By making small but impactful changes to your lifestyle, you can transform your heart health and reduce your risk of heart disease. The power of self-care lies in your hands, and by prioritizing your well-being, you are taking a proactive step towards a healthier heart and a longer, happier life.

Remember, you have the ability to make a difference in your heart health. Start today by implementing these lifestyle medicine principles and witness the transformative power of self-care in your life.

How Poor Lifestyle Habits Contribute to Heart Problems

Introduction:

In our modern society, heart problems have become increasingly prevalent, affecting people from all walks of life. While genetic factors play a role, it is important to recognize the significant impact that poor lifestyle habits have on heart health. This subchapter explores the various ways in which our choices and habits can contribute to heart problems. By understanding these connections, we can empower ourselves to make positive changes and prioritize self-care for heart health using lifestyle medicine principles.

Sedentary Lifestyle:

One major factor contributing to heart problems is a sedentary lifestyle. As technology advances, physical activity decreases, leading to weight gain, high blood pressure, and increased cholesterol levels. By sitting for long periods and neglecting regular exercise, we put ourselves at a higher risk of developing heart disease.

Unhealthy Diet:

The food we consume has a profound impact on our heart health. A diet high in saturated and trans fats, processed foods, sugary beverages, and excessive sodium can lead to obesity, high blood pressure, and elevated cholesterol levels. Poor dietary choices contribute to inflammation, insulin resistance, and the accumulation of plaque in the arteries, increasing the risk of heart problems.

Smoking and Excessive Alcohol Consumption:

Smoking and excessive alcohol consumption are detrimental to heart health. Cigarette smoke damages blood vessels, reduces oxygen supply, and increases the risk of blood clots. Similarly, excessive alcohol intake can lead to high blood pressure, irregular heart rhythms, and weaken heart muscles. Quitting smoking and moderating alcohol consumption are crucial steps in improving heart health.

Chronic Stress:

Stress has a profound effect on our overall well-being, including heart health. Chronic stress increases blood pressure, elevates heart rate, and promotes the release of stress hormones, all of which contribute to the development of heart problems. Incorporating stress management techniques such as meditation, yoga, and regular relaxation can significantly reduce the risk.

Conclusion:

It is clear that poor lifestyle habits significantly contribute to heart problems. Recognizing the impact of a sedentary lifestyle, unhealthy diet, smoking, excessive alcohol consumption, and chronic stress on heart health is the first step towards change. By embracing self-care principles rooted in lifestyle medicine, we can transform our heart health and reduce the risk of heart problems. Through regular physical activity, a balanced and nutritious diet, quitting harmful habits, and managing stress effectively, we empower ourselves to take control of our heart health and live a healthier, more fulfilling life.

The Benefits of Adopting a Healthy Lifestyle

In today's fast-paced world, it's easy to neglect our health amidst our busy schedules and demanding responsibilities. However, taking care of our well-being should be a top priority, especially when it comes to heart health. Adopting a healthy lifestyle can significantly improve our overall well-being and reduce the risk of heart disease. In this subchapter, we will explore the numerous benefits of incorporating self-care for heart health using lifestyle medicine principles.

First and foremost, adopting a healthy lifestyle can enhance our cardiovascular health. Regular physical activity, such as brisk walking, jogging, or cycling, strengthens our heart muscles and improves blood circulation. Engaging in these activities not only helps to maintain a healthy weight but also lowers blood pressure and cholesterol levels. By making exercise a part of our daily routine, we can significantly reduce the risk of heart disease and other related conditions.

Furthermore, healthy eating plays a crucial role in maintaining heart health. A diet rich in fruits, vegetables, whole grains, and lean proteins provides essential nutrients and antioxidants that protect our heart and blood vessels. By avoiding processed foods high in saturated fats, trans fats, and excessive salt, we can lower cholesterol levels and keep our blood pressure in check. Adopting a heart-healthy diet not only improves our cardiovascular health but also benefits our overall well-being.

In addition to exercise and a healthy diet, managing stress and practicing self-care are vital components of a healthy lifestyle. Chronic stress can have a detrimental impact on our heart health, increasing the risk of heart disease and heart attacks. Engaging in stress-reducing activities such as meditation, yoga, or spending quality time with loved ones can help lower stress levels and improve heart health.

Lastly, quitting harmful habits like smoking and excessive alcohol consumption significantly reduces the risk of heart disease. Smoking damages blood vessels and increases the likelihood of developing atherosclerosis, while excessive alcohol consumption can lead to high blood pressure and heart failure. By adopting a healthy lifestyle and eliminating these harmful habits, we can greatly improve our heart health and overall well-being.

In conclusion, adopting a healthy lifestyle and practicing self-care is essential for maintaining heart health. By incorporating regular exercise, healthy eating, stress management, and quitting harmful habits, we can significantly reduce the risk of heart disease and enjoy a higher quality of life. It's never too late to prioritize our well-being and make positive changes that will benefit our hearts for years to come.

03

Self-Care Practices for a Healthy Heart

Nutrition and Heart Health

Proper nutrition plays a crucial role in maintaining a healthy heart and preventing various cardiovascular diseases. In this subchapter, we will explore the significant impact of nutrition on heart health and how following lifestyle medicine principles can help promote self-care in this regard.

A well-balanced diet rich in nutrients is essential for maintaining optimal heart health. Consuming a variety of fruits, vegetables, whole grains, lean proteins, and healthy fats can provide the necessary nutrients to support heart function and reduce the risk of heart disease. These foods are low in saturated and trans fats, cholesterol, sodium, and added sugars, which are known contributors to heart problems.

One important aspect of nutrition for heart health is understanding the role of macronutrients. Carbohydrates, proteins, and fats are the three main macronutrients that our bodies need in varying amounts. Choosing the right types and proportions of these macronutrients is crucial. For instance, opting for complex carbohydrates like whole grains instead of refined carbohydrates can help regulate blood sugar levels and reduce the risk of diabetes, which is a major risk factor for heart disease.

Furthermore, consuming lean proteins such as fish, poultry, and legumes instead of red meat can help lower cholesterol levels and maintain a healthy weight. Healthy fats, such as those found in avocados, nuts, and olive oil, are essential for heart health as they can help lower bad cholesterol levels and reduce inflammation.

Moreover, it is important to be mindful of portion sizes and practice moderation in our eating habits. Overeating can lead to weight gain, obesity, and other risk factors for heart disease. Incorporating mindful eating practices, such as eating slowly and paying attention to hunger and fullness cues, can help promote self-care and prevent overeating.

In addition to choosing the right foods, it is crucial to stay hydrated for optimal heart health. Drinking an adequate amount of water throughout the day helps maintain blood viscosity, prevents dehydration, and promotes overall cardiovascular health.

In conclusion, nutrition plays a vital role in maintaining heart health. By following lifestyle medicine principles, including consuming a well- balanced diet rich in fruits, vegetables, whole grains, lean proteins, and healthy fats, individuals can promote self-care for their heart health. Being mindful of portion sizes and staying hydrated are equally important for maintaining optimal cardiovascular well-being. By making these dietary changes, anyone can take proactive steps towards transforming their heart health and embracing a lifestyle that supports overall well- being.

The Heart-Healthy Diet: What to Eat and What to Avoid

When it comes to maintaining a healthy heart, following a well-balanced diet is crucial. The food we eat plays a significant role in our overall heart health, and making smart choices can greatly reduce the risk of heart disease. In this subchapter, we will explore the key principles of a heart-healthy diet, including what to eat and what to avoid.

Eating a variety of nutrient-rich foods is at the core of a heart-healthy diet. Filling your plate with fruits, vegetables, whole grains, and lean proteins can provide essential vitamins, minerals, and fiber that support heart health. Incorporating colorful fruits and vegetables ensures a wide range of antioxidants, which protect against oxidative stress and inflammation. Whole grains like brown rice, quinoa, and whole wheat bread provide complex carbohydrates and fiber, while lean proteins such as fish, poultry, and legumes offer essential amino acids without the excess saturated fats found in red meats.

Omega-3 fatty acids, found in fatty fish like salmon, mackerel, and sardines, are particularly beneficial for heart health. These healthy fats help lower blood pressure and reduce the risk of abnormal heart rhythms. Including a serving of fatty fish in your diet at least twice a week can have a profound impact on your heart health.

On the other hand, there are certain foods that should be limited or avoided to maintain a heart-healthy diet. These include foods high in saturated and trans fats, sodium, and added sugars. Saturated fats, commonly found in red meats, full-fat dairy products, and processed foods, can raise cholesterol levels and increase the risk of heart disease. Trans fats, often found in fried and commercially baked goods, should be completely avoided as they not only raise bad cholesterol but also lower good cholesterol.

Additionally, excessive sodium intake can contribute to high blood pressure, a major risk factor for heart disease. Limiting sodium consumption by reducing processed and packaged foods, and opting for fresh ingredients, can significantly improve heart health. Similarly, cutting back on added sugars found in sugary beverages, desserts, and sweetened snacks can help maintain a healthy weight and prevent conditions such as obesity and diabetes, which are closely linked to heart disease.

By adopting a heart-healthy diet, you can take control of your heart health and reduce the risk of cardiovascular diseases. Incorporating nutrient-rich foods, limiting saturated and trans fats, reducing sodium intake, and avoiding added sugars are essential steps towards transforming your heart health with lifestyle medicine principles. Remember, every small dietary change can make a big difference in the long run. Start today and prioritize your heart health through the power of self-care.

The Role of Macronutrients in Maintaining Heart Health

The Role of Macronutrients in Maintaining Heart Health

When it comes to maintaining heart health, focusing on macronutrients is crucial. Macronutrients are the nutrients that our bodies need in large quantities, namely carbohydrates, proteins, and fats. These nutrients play a significant role in providing energy, building and repairing tissues, and supporting various bodily functions. By understanding the role of macronutrients in maintaining heart health, we can make informed choices about our diet and embrace self-care practices for a healthier heart.

Carbohydrates are the primary source of energy for our bodies. They are found in foods such as grains, fruits, vegetables, and legumes. Choosing complex carbohydrates, such as whole grains and fiber-rich foods, is beneficial for heart health. These carbohydrates are digested slowly, preventing spikes in blood sugar levels and reducing the risk of developing conditions like diabetes, which can negatively impact heart health.

Proteins are essential for repairing and building tissues, including the heart muscles. Lean sources of protein, such as poultry, fish, legumes, and low-fat dairy products, are recommended for a heart-healthy diet. These protein sources are low in saturated fats, which can raise cholesterol levels and increase the risk of heart disease. Including plant-based proteins, like beans and lentils, can further promote heart health by reducing the consumption of animal-based saturated fats.

Fats are often associated with negative health effects, but not all fats are created equal. Unsaturated fats, found in foods like avocados, nuts, seeds, and olive oil, are heart-healthy fats that can help reduce bad cholesterol levels and lower the risk of heart disease. On the other hand, saturated and trans fats, commonly found in processed foods, fried foods, and fatty meats, should be limited as they can raise cholesterol levels and contribute to heart disease.

Incorporating a balanced mix of macronutrients into our diets is vital for maintaining heart health. A diet rich in whole grains, fruits, vegetables, lean proteins, and healthy fats can provide the necessary nutrients to support heart function and reduce the risk of heart disease. It is essential to focus on portion control and mindful eating to maintain a healthy weight, which is another crucial aspect of heart health.

By understanding the role of macronutrients and making conscious choices about our diet, we can embrace self-care practices that promote heart health using lifestyle medicine principles. Taking charge of our diet and incorporating heart-healthy macronutrients can significantly impact our overall well-being and reduce the risk of cardiovascular diseases. Remember, small changes in our eating habits can lead to significant improvements in heart health, making self-care a powerful tool in transforming our lives.

Incorporating Superfoods for Optimal Heart Function

When it comes to maintaining a healthy heart, there is no doubt that diet plays a crucial role. The food we consume has a direct impact on our heart health, and incorporating superfoods into our daily meals can be a game-changer. Superfoods are not only packed with essential nutrients but also possess unique properties that promote optimal heart function. In this subchapter, we will explore how incorporating superfoods can transform your heart health and enhance your overall well-being.

One superfood that stands out in promoting heart health is salmon. Rich in omega-3 fatty acids, salmon has been proven to reduce the risk of heart disease and lower cholesterol levels. By incorporating this fatty fish into your diet at least twice a week, you can significantly improve your heart health. Other sources of omega-3 fatty acids include chia seeds, flaxseeds, and walnuts, which can be easily added to your meals or enjoyed as snacks.

Berries, such as blueberries, strawberries, and raspberries, are another group of superfoods that promote heart health. Packed with antioxidants and fiber, berries help reduce inflammation, lower blood pressure, and improve overall cardiovascular function. Adding a handful of berries to your morning oatmeal or yogurt can be a simple yet effective way to incorporate these superfoods into your diet.

Leafy greens, such as spinach and kale, are also essential for heart health. These greens are rich in vitamins, minerals, and antioxidants that protect against heart disease. They are also low in calories, making them a great addition to any weight management plan. Whether in salads, smoothies, or sautéed as a side dish, leafy greens should be a staple in your diet for optimal heart function.

In addition to these superfoods, incorporating dark chocolate, green tea, and nuts like almonds and walnuts into your diet can provide further benefits to your heart health. Dark chocolate has been shown to improve blood flow and reduce the risk of blood clots, while green tea helps lower cholesterol levels and blood pressure. Nuts, on the other hand, are rich in healthy fats, fiber, and antioxidants that promote heart health.

By incorporating these superfoods into your daily meals, you can transform your heart health and overall well-being. Remember, self-care for heart health using lifestyle medicine principles begins with the choices we make in our diet. Start making these small changes today, and witness the powerful impact they can have on your heart health.

Physical Activity and Heart Health

Physical activity plays a crucial role in maintaining a healthy heart and overall well-being. In this subchapter, we will explore the significant impact of regular exercise on heart health and how it can be incorporated into your daily self-care routine using lifestyle medicine principles.

Engaging in physical activity is one of the most effective ways to reduce the risk of heart disease. Regular exercise helps strengthen the heart muscle, improves blood circulation, and lowers blood pressure, cholesterol levels, and the risk of developing diabetes. It also aids in maintaining a healthy weight, which is vital for heart health.

The benefits of physical activity extend beyond the heart. Exercise enhances mental health, reduces stress, boosts mood, and improves overall quality of life. It promotes better sleep, increases energy levels, and enhances cognitive function. By incorporating physical activity into your daily routine, you are not only taking care of your heart but also nurturing your mind and body.

When it comes to self-care for heart health using lifestyle medicine principles, it is important to find activities that you enjoy and can sustain in the long run. This could include brisk walking, jogging, swimming, cycling, or even dancing. The key is to engage in moderate-intensity aerobic exercise for at least 150 minutes per week or vigorous-intensity exercise for 75 minutes per week, spread across several days.

It is also beneficial to incorporate strength training exercises into your routine at least twice a week. These exercises help build muscle mass, improve metabolism, and enhance overall physical performance. Additionally, flexibility and balance exercises such as yoga or Tai Chi can improve posture, prevent injuries, and promote relaxation.

To get started, it is advisable to consult with your healthcare provider, especially if you have any existing health conditions or if you have been leading a sedentary lifestyle. They can provide personalized recommendations and guidance based on your individual needs and health status.

In conclusion, physical activity is a powerful tool for maintaining heart health and overall well-being. By incorporating regular exercise into your daily routine, you can significantly reduce the risk of heart disease, improve mental health, and enhance your quality of life. Remember, self- care for heart health using lifestyle medicine principles is about making conscious choices to prioritize your well-being and taking the necessary steps to maintain a healthy heart.

The Importance of Regular Exercise for a Healthy Heart

Exercise is often touted as one of the most powerful tools for maintaining a healthy heart. It plays a pivotal role in preventing heart disease and promoting overall cardiovascular health. In this subchapter, we will explore the significance of regular exercise in safeguarding your heart and discuss how incorporating physical activity into your daily routine can transform your heart health.

Physical inactivity is a leading risk factor for heart disease. Sedentary lifestyles have become increasingly common in our modern society, with advancements in technology and a shift towards more sedentary jobs. However, our bodies were designed to move, and regular exercise is essential for maintaining optimal heart health.

Engaging in regular physical activity offers a myriad of benefits for your heart. First and foremost, exercise helps to strengthen the heart muscle, making it more efficient at pumping blood throughout the body. This increased efficiency reduces the strain on the heart, lowering the risk of developing various cardiovascular diseases, including heart attacks and strokes.

Exercise also plays a crucial role in maintaining a healthy weight, which is vital for heart health. Regular physical activity helps to burn calories and build lean muscle, contributing to weight management. Maintaining a healthy weight reduces the risk of developing conditions such as high blood pressure, high cholesterol, and diabetes, which are all major contributors to heart disease.

Furthermore, exercise has been shown to improve blood circulation and reduce inflammation, both of which are key factors in maintaining a healthy cardiovascular system. By increasing blood flow, exercise helps to deliver oxygen and nutrients to the heart and other organs, promoting their proper functioning. Additionally, regular physical activity stimulates the release of endorphins, also known as the "feel-good" hormones, which can help reduce stress and improve overall mental well-being.

Incorporating exercise into your daily routine doesn't have to be overwhelming. Start by setting realistic goals and gradually increase the intensity and duration of your workouts. Aim for at least 150 minutes of moderate-intensity aerobic exercise, such as brisk walking or cycling, every week, along with muscle-strengthening activities at least twice a week.

Remember, self-care for heart health using lifestyle medicine principles is all about making sustainable changes that can be maintained in the long run. Regular exercise is a cornerstone of this approach, providing numerous benefits for your heart and overall well-being. By prioritizing physical activity and incorporating it into your daily life, you can transform your heart health and enjoy a healthier, happier life.

Types of Exercises that Promote Heart Health

Regular physical activity is crucial for maintaining a healthy heart and preventing cardiovascular diseases. In this subchapter, we will explore various types of exercises that promote heart health and can be incorporated into your self-care routine using lifestyle medicine principles.

Aerobic Exercises: Also known as cardio exercises, these activities increase your heart rate and help strengthen your heart. Examples include brisk walking, jogging, swimming, cycling, and dancing. Aim for at least 150 minutes of moderate-intensity aerobic activity or 75 minutes of vigorous-intensity aerobic activity per week, or a combination of both.

Strength Training: Incorporating strength training exercises into your routine helps build lean muscle mass, which boosts metabolism and improves overall cardiovascular health. Engage in activities like weightlifting, using resistance bands, or doing bodyweight exercises such as push-ups, squats, and lunges. Aim for two or more days of strength training exercises per week, targeting major muscle groups.

High-Intensity Interval Training (HIIT): HIIT involves short bursts of intense exercise followed by brief recovery periods. This type of exercise helps improve cardiovascular fitness and can be customized to suit various fitness levels. Examples of HIIT workouts include sprint intervals, circuit training, or Tabata workouts. Start with short intervals and gradually increase the intensity and duration as your fitness improves.

Flexibility Exercises: Stretching exercises enhance flexibility, improve circulation, and reduce muscle tension. Incorporate activities like yoga, Pilates, or simple stretching routines into your weekly exercise plan. Focus on stretching major muscle groups, holding each stretch for 10-30 seconds without bouncing.

Balance Training: Maintaining good balance is essential for preventing falls, especially as we age. Balance exercises can be as simple as standing on one leg or more advanced, involving yoga poses like tree pose or warrior stance. Include balance exercises in your routine at least two days per week.

Remember, before starting any exercise program, it is essential to consult with your healthcare provider, especially if you have pre-existing heart conditions or any other health concerns. They can provide personalized recommendations based on your fitness level and medical history.

Incorporating these types of exercises into your self-care routine can significantly improve your heart health. Start slowly, and gradually increase the intensity and duration of your workouts. Remember to listen to your body and adapt the exercises to suit your fitness level. Consistency is key, so aim for regular physical activity to maximize the benefits for your heart and overall well-being.

Developing a Personalized Exercise Routine for Heart Health

Exercise is a crucial component of maintaining a healthy heart. It not only strengthens the cardiovascular system but also helps manage weight, reduce stress, and improve overall well-being. However, not all exercise routines are created equal, and it is essential to develop a personalized plan that suits your specific needs and goals. This subchapter will guide you through the process of creating an exercise routine tailored to promote heart health using lifestyle medicine principles.

Before embarking on any exercise program, it is crucial to consult with your healthcare provider to ensure it aligns with your current health status. Once you have the green light, it's time to start designing your personalized exercise routine.

Begin by assessing your current fitness level. Consider factors such as your age, weight, and overall health. This self-evaluation will help you determine the intensity and duration of exercise that is appropriate for you. If you are new to exercise or have any underlying health conditions, it may be best to start with low-impact activities such as walking or swimming and gradually increase the intensity over time.

Next, identify your goals. Are you looking to lose weight, lower blood pressure, or simply enhance your cardiovascular fitness? Setting clear objectives will help you stay motivated and track your progress. Remember to be realistic and focus on gradual improvements rather than expecting instant results.

Once you have determined your goals, it's time to choose the right type of exercise. Aim for a combination of aerobic activities, strength training, and flexibility exercises. Aerobic exercises, such as brisk walking or cycling, increase your heart rate and strengthen your heart. Incorporating strength training exercises, such as lifting weights or using resistance bands, helps build muscle mass, which in turn improves heart health. Finally, don't forget about flexibility exercises, such as yoga or stretching, which enhance mobility and prevent injuries.

Create a weekly exercise schedule that includes a variety of activities to keep you engaged and prevent boredom. Aim for at least 150 minutes of moderate-intensity aerobic activity or 75 minutes of vigorous-intensity aerobic activity per week, spread out across several days. Additionally, incorporate strength training at least two days a week, targeting major muscle groups.

Remember to listen to your body and make adjustments as needed. If you experience any pain or discomfort during exercise, modify or stop the activity and consult with your healthcare provider.

By developing a personalized exercise routine focused on heart health, you can take control of your well-being and improve your quality of life. Regular exercise, combined with other lifestyle medicine principles such as a healthy diet and stress management techniques, has the power to transform your heart health and promote overall wellness.

Stress Management and Heart Health

In today's fast-paced and demanding world, stress has become an unavoidable part of our lives. From work pressures to personal responsibilities, stress can take a toll on our overall well-being, especially our heart health. However, by adopting effective stress management techniques, we can significantly improve our heart health and overall quality of life.

Stress, if left unchecked, can have a detrimental impact on our cardiovascular system. When we are stressed, our body releases stress hormones like cortisol and adrenaline, which can elevate blood pressure and increase heart rate. Prolonged exposure to stress can lead to chronic inflammation, arterial damage, and an increased risk of heart disease.

Fortunately, incorporating self-care practices using lifestyle medicine principles can help manage and reduce stress, subsequently improving heart health. Here are some strategies to consider:

Exercise: Engaging in regular physical activity is a powerful stress reliever. Exercise releases endorphins, which act as natural mood boosters and reduce stress levels. Aim for at least 30 minutes of moderate-intensity exercise, such as brisk walking or cycling, most days of the week.

Mindfulness and Meditation: Practicing mindfulness and meditation techniques can help calm the mind, reduce anxiety, and promote relaxation. Set aside a few minutes each day to focus on your breath, observe your thoughts without judgment, and cultivate a sense of inner peace.

Healthy Diet: Nourishing your body with a heart-healthy diet can also combat stress. Incorporate plenty of fruits, vegetables, whole grains, lean proteins, and healthy fats into your meals. Limit your intake of processed foods, sugary snacks, and excessive caffeine, as these can exacerbate stress responses.

Quality Sleep: Adequate sleep is crucial for stress management and heart health. Establish a consistent sleep routine, create a relaxing sleep environment, and aim for 7-8 hours of quality sleep each night.

Social Support: Surrounding yourself with a strong support system can help alleviate stress. Cultivate meaningful relationships, engage in positive social interactions, and seek support from loved ones during challenging times.

By prioritizing self-care practices and incorporating these lifestyle medicine principles into our daily lives, we can effectively manage stress and improve our heart health. Remember, self-care is not a luxury; it is an essential investment in our overall well-being. Take the time to nurture your heart, and it will reward you with better health and vitality.

Understanding the Relationship Between Stress and Heart Disease

In today's fast-paced and demanding world, stress has become an inevitable part of our lives. From work pressures to personal challenges, we all experience stress at some point. While it is normal to feel stressed occasionally, chronic and unmanaged stress can have severe consequences on our overall health, particularly our heart health. This subchapter aims to shed light on the intricate relationship between stress and heart disease and provide valuable insights into practicing self-care for heart health using lifestyle medicine principles.

Stress, when left unchecked, can wreak havoc on our cardiovascular system. The body's response to stress involves the release of stress hormones like cortisol and adrenaline, which can increase blood pressure, heart rate, and cause inflammation. These physiological changes, when prolonged, can lead to the development of various heart conditions such as hypertension, atherosclerosis, and even heart attacks.

It is crucial to recognize the signs of stress and its impact on our heart health. Symptoms like chest pain, rapid heartbeat, fatigue, and difficulty sleeping should not be ignored, as they could be early warning signs of heart disease. By understanding the relationship between stress and heart health, we can take proactive measures to manage stress and protect our hearts.

Lifestyle medicine principles offer a holistic approach to self-care for heart health. Through simple yet effective lifestyle modifications, we can significantly reduce stress levels and promote a healthier heart. Regular exercise, for instance, not only helps to relieve stress but also improves cardiovascular fitness. Engaging in activities like yoga, meditation, or deep breathing exercises can also calm the mind and reduce stress levels.

Furthermore, adopting a healthy diet rich in fruits, vegetables, whole grains, and lean proteins can provide essential nutrients that support heart health. Avoiding excessive caffeine, alcohol, and processed foods is equally important. Adequate sleep is another crucial aspect of self- care for heart health, as it allows the body to recover from daily stressors and maintain optimal cardiovascular function.

In conclusion, understanding the relationship between stress and heart disease is paramount in our journey towards optimal heart health. By implementing lifestyle medicine principles and practicing self-care, we can effectively manage stress levels and protect our hearts from the detrimental effects of chronic stress. Empowering ourselves with knowledge and taking proactive steps towards a healthier lifestyle is the key to transforming our heart health and living a fulfilling life. Remember, self-care is not a luxury but a necessity when it comes to nurturing our hearts and overall well-being.

Effective Techniques for Stress Reduction

Effective Techniques for Stress Reduction

Stress has become an inevitable part of our modern lifestyle, affecting people from all walks of life. Whether you're a busy professional, a stay- at-home parent, or a student juggling multiple responsibilities, stress can take a toll on your overall well-being, particularly your heart health. In this subchapter, we will explore some effective techniques for stress reduction that can help you transform your heart health using the principles of lifestyle medicine.

1. Deep Breathing: One of the simplest yet most powerful techniques for stress reduction is deep breathing. By taking slow, deep breaths, you activate the body's relaxation response, which helps to calm your mind and reduce stress levels. Find a quiet place, sit comfortably, and take a deep breath in through your nose, allowing your abdomen to expand. Then exhale slowly through your mouth, focusing on releasing any tension or worry. Repeat this process for a few minutes each day, especially during times of heightened stress.

Practice the following deep breathing techniques:

- Diaphragmatic breathing: Place one hand on your abdomen and inhale deeply through your nose, allowing your belly to rise. Exhale slowly through your mouth, letting your belly fall. Repeat this pattern, gently focusing on the sensation of your breath.

- Box breathing: Inhale deeply for a count of four, hold your breath for a count of four, exhale for a count of four, and hold for a count of four. Repeat this cycle multiple times, visualizing a box shape with each breath

2. Mindfulness Meditation: Practicing mindfulness meditation can have transformative effects on your stress levels and heart health. By focusing your attention on the present moment, without judgment or attachment, you can cultivate a sense of calm and reduce the impact of stress on your body. Set aside a few minutes each day to sit quietly, close your eyes, and bring your attention to your breath or a specific focal point. As thoughts arise, simply observe them without getting caught up in their content, and gently shift your focus back to the present moment.

Mindfulness allows us to fully experience each moment, fostering a greater sense of gratitude and contentment. Mindfulness can be practiced through activities such as meditation, yoga, or even while engaging in everyday tasks like eating or walking. By being fully present, we can reduce anxiety, improve focus, and cultivate a deeper connection with ourselves and others.

Incorporate mindfulness techniques into your daily routine:

- Body scan meditation: Lie down or sit in a comfortable position, and slowly bring your attention to distinct parts of your body, scanning for any sensations or tension. Allow yourself to relax and release any tension you may feel.

- Guided imagery: Engage in guided visualization exercises, where you imagine yourself in a peaceful and calming environment. Picture yourself in a serene location, such as a beach or forest, and focus on the sensory details, such as the sound of waves or the smell of nature

Using yoga and gentle stretching for relaxation

Engage in gentle yoga or stretching exercises to release tension from your body and promote relaxation. Yoga combines physical movements, breathing techniques, and meditation, making it an excellent stress-reducing activity. Engaging in yoga or gentle stretching exercises can help release physical tension and calm the mind.

Consider the following practices:

- Hatha yoga: Hatha yoga focuses on gentle poses and slow movements, allowing you to connect with your breath and release tension. Attend yoga classes or follow online tutorials specifically designed for relaxation and stress reduction.

- Restorative yoga: Restorative yoga involves using props, such as bolsters and blankets, to support your body in relaxing poses for an extended period. This practice encourages deep relaxation and rejuvenation.

Find activities that help you relax and promote a positive mindset.

Consider engaging in activities such as:

- Listening to soothing music: Create a playlist of calming music or nature sounds that help you relax and unwind. Listening to pleasant music can have a positive impact on your mood and reduce stress levels.

- Engaging in creative outlets: Explore creative outlets such as painting, writing, or playing a musical instrument. These activities can serve as a form of self-expression and supply a therapeutic escape from stressors.

- Spending time in nature: Spend time outdoors in natural environments, such as parks or gardens. Connecting with nature and being outdoors has been shown to reduce stress, boost your mood, and promote overall well-being

3. Physical Activity: Regular physical activity not only improves heart health but also serves as a powerful stress reducer. Engaging in activities such as brisk walking, jogging, dancing, or yoga releases endorphins, the brain's natural mood boosters, which help combat stress and promote a sense of well-being. Aim for at least 30 minutes of moderate intensity exercise most days of the week, and choose activities that you enjoy to make it a sustainable habit.

4. Sleep Hygiene: Adequate sleep is essential for managing stress and maintaining heart health. Establishing a regular sleep routine, avoiding excessive caffeine and electronic device use before bed, and creating a comfortable sleep environment can significantly improve the quality and duration of your sleep. Aim for 7-8 hours of uninterrupted sleep each night to give your body the rest it needs to recover from daily stressors.

Incorporating relaxation and mindfulness practices into our daily lives doesn't have to be complicated or time-consuming. It can be as simple as taking a few minutes each day to engage in deep breathing exercises or setting aside a specific time for meditation or yoga practice. By making these practices a priority, we can create a positive shift in our mindset and overall well-being.

Moreover, it is important to remember that self-care is not selfish; it is an essential component of maintaining heart health. By prioritizing relaxation and mindfulness, we are taking proactive steps towards caring for ourselves, reducing the risk of heart disease, and enhancing our overall quality of life.

In conclusion, incorporating relaxation and mindfulness practices into our daily lives is a powerful tool in self-care for heart health. By taking the time to engage in these practices, we can reduce stress, improve our overall well-being, and create a stronger connection with ourselves. So, why wait? Start incorporating relaxation and mindfulness practices into your daily routine today and experience the transformative power of self-care for heart health.

Sleep and Heart Health

Sleep is a fundamental aspect of our daily lives, yet it is often overlooked when it comes to heart health. Many people prioritize diet and exercise but fail to realize the significant impact that sleep can have on their overall well-being, particularly when it comes to the health of their heart. In this subchapter, we will explore the vital connection between sleep and heart health, and how incorporating proper sleep practices into your self-care routine can help transform your heart health using lifestyle medicine principles.

Research has shown that inadequate sleep can have detrimental effects on cardiovascular health. Lack of sleep has been linked to an increased risk of developing conditions such as high blood pressure, heart disease, and stroke. When we sleep, our bodies undergo essential processes that help regulate blood pressure, reduce inflammation, and maintain a healthy balance of hormones. Without enough sleep, these crucial functions are disrupted, putting undue stress on our hearts.

Furthermore, poor sleep quality has been associated with an increased risk of obesity and diabetes, both of which are significant risk factors for heart disease. Sleep deprivation can disrupt the balance of hunger-regulating hormones, leading to increased appetite and cravings for unhealthy foods. It can also impair glucose metabolism, leading to insulin resistance and elevated blood sugar levels. By prioritizing quality sleep, we can effectively manage these risk factors and promote a healthier heart.

So how can we improve our sleep and promote optimal heart health? Firstly, it is important to establish a regular sleep schedule, ensuring that we are getting an adequate amount of sleep each night. Most adults require between seven to nine hours of sleep for optimal functioning. Additionally, creating a relaxing bedtime routine can help signal the body that it is time to wind down. This can include activities such as reading, taking a warm bath, or practicing relaxation techniques like deep breathing or meditation.

Creating a sleep-friendly environment is also essential. Ensure that your bedroom is dark, quiet, and at a comfortable temperature. Limit exposure to electronic devices before bed, as the blue light emitted can interfere with your sleep-wake cycle. Finally, avoid consuming stimulating substances like caffeine or nicotine close to bedtime, as they can disrupt your ability to fall asleep.

In conclusion, sleep plays a crucial role in maintaining heart health. By prioritizing quality sleep and incorporating proper sleep practices into our self-care routine, we can significantly reduce the risk of developing cardiovascular conditions. Remember, self-care for heart health goes beyond diet and exercise – adequate sleep is a vital component of a comprehensive lifestyle medicine approach. So take the time to invest in your sleep, and watch as your heart health transforms for the better.

The Impact of Sleep on Heart Function

Sleep is an essential component of our daily lives, contributing to our overall health and well-being. It is during sleep that our bodies undergo crucial processes for rejuvenation, repair, and restoration. While it is commonly known that sleep plays a vital role in mental and physical health, its impact on heart function is often overlooked. In this subchapter, we will explore the profound influence that sleep has on our heart health and how prioritizing quality sleep can transform our cardiovascular well-being.

The connection between sleep and heart function is multifaceted. Research has consistently demonstrated that inadequate or poor-quality sleep can have detrimental effects on our cardiovascular system. One of the key mechanisms behind this is the disruption of the body's natural circadian rhythm. Our internal clock, regulated by the sleep-wake cycle, helps maintain the balance of various physiological processes, including heart rate, blood pressure, and hormone production. When this rhythm is disrupted due to insufficient sleep, it can lead to increased blood pressure, irregular heart rhythms, and a higher risk of developing heart disease.

Furthermore, sleep deprivation has been linked to an increased prevalence of obesity, diabetes, and metabolic syndrome, all of which are significant risk factors for cardiovascular disease. Lack of sleep alters the hormones that regulate hunger and satiety, leading to increased appetite and cravings for high-calorie foods. This can contribute to weight gain and the development of conditions that negatively impact heart health.

On the other hand, prioritizing adequate and quality sleep can have profound benefits for our heart. Studies have shown that individuals who consistently get enough sleep have lower blood pressure, reduced inflammation, and a decreased risk of heart disease. Additionally, quality sleep promotes the body's natural healing processes, allowing for better recovery from daily stressors and improving overall cardiovascular function.

Incorporating self-care practices that prioritize sleep hygiene into our daily routines can be transformative for our heart health. Establishing a consistent sleep schedule, creating a sleep-friendly environment, and adopting relaxation techniques can all contribute to improved sleep quality. Additionally, avoiding stimulants such as caffeine and electronic devices before bedtime can help regulate our body's natural sleep-wake cycle.

In conclusion, sleep plays a critical role in maintaining optimal heart function. By recognizing the impact of sleep on our cardiovascular well-being and prioritizing quality sleep through self-care practices, we can significantly transform our heart health. Investing in adequate sleep is a powerful lifestyle medicine principle that can contribute to a healthier, happier heart.

Establishing Healthy Sleep Habits for Heart Health

Sleep plays a crucial role in maintaining overall well-being, and its impact on heart health cannot be underestimated. In this subchapter, we will explore the significance of healthy sleep habits in promoting heart health and how lifestyle medicine principles can be used for effective self- care.

Sleep deprivation has become a common problem in today's fast-paced society, with many individuals sacrificing sleep to meet various demands in their lives. However, research has consistently shown that inadequate sleep can have detrimental effects on cardiovascular health. Lack of sleep has been linked to an increased risk of developing conditions such as hypertension, obesity, diabetes, and even heart disease.

To establish healthy sleep habits, it is important to prioritize and allocate sufficient time for sleep. Aim for seven to nine hours of uninterrupted sleep each night. Create a calming sleep environment by keeping your bedroom cool, dark, and quiet. Avoid exposure to electronic devices before bed, as the blue light emitted from screens can disrupt your natural sleep-wake cycle.

Developing a bedtime routine can also greatly improve sleep quality. Engage in relaxing activities such as reading a book, practicing meditation or deep breathing exercises, or taking a warm bath. Consistency is key, as sticking to a regular sleep schedule can help regulate your body's internal clock and improve sleep efficiency.

Incorporating lifestyle medicine principles into your self-care routine can further enhance the benefits of healthy sleep habits for heart health. Regular exercise has been proven to promote better sleep quality. Engage in aerobic activities such as brisk walking, swimming, or cycling for at least 150 minutes per week. However, avoid vigorous exercise close to bedtime, as it may stimulate your body and make it difficult to fall asleep.

Dietary choices also play a crucial role in sleep quality and heart health. Avoid consuming large meals, caffeine, or alcohol close to bedtime, as they can disrupt sleep patterns. Instead, opt for a light snack that includes sleep-promoting nutrients such as magnesium, tryptophan, and calcium. Incorporate foods like bananas, almonds, and leafy greens into your evening routine. Establishing a sleep routine

Creating a consistent sleep routine is essential for promoting quality sleep and maximizing your overall well-being before surgery. We will now explore the steps you can take to set up a healthy sleep routine.

Focus on creating a relaxing bedtime routine: A bedtime routine helps signal to your body that it's time to unwind and prepare for sleep. By engaging in calming activities before bed, you can promote relaxation and optimize your chances of falling asleep more easily.

- Avoid using electronic devices: Minimise exposure to devices, such as smartphones, tablets, or laptops, at least an hour before bedtime. The blue light emitted by these devices can interfere with your sleep by suppressing the production of melatonin, a hormone that regulates sleep.

- Set up a wind-down period: Engage in activities that promote relaxation, such as reading a book, listening to soothing music, practicing gentle stretching or yoga, taking a warm bath, or practicing mindfulness or meditation techniques.

- Create consistency: Perform your bedtime routine in the same order and at approximately the same time each night to establish a consistent pattern that signals to your body that it's time to sleep. Consider using blue light blocking glasses in the hours before bed.

Choose activities that you find personally enjoyable and that help you relax and unwind. Experiment with different relaxation techniques to find what works best for you. Be consistent and make your bedtime routine a priority every night.

Creating a sleep-friendly environment: This can significantly enhance the quality of your sleep. By optimising your sleep environment, you can minimize potential disturbances and create a space that promotes restful sleep.

- Darkness: Use blackout curtains or an eye mask to block out external light sources that may disrupt your sleep. Consider using a dim night light if you need to navigate your bedroom during the night.

- Noise control: Use earplugs, a white noise machine, or a fan to mask disruptive noises and create a soothing background sound.

- Temperature and comfort: Keep your bedroom well-ventilated, and at a temperature that is conducive to sleep. Use comfortable bedding, pillows, and mattresses that support your body's needs.

Remove electronic devices and other potential distractions from your bedroom. Make sure your mattress and pillows supply adequate support and comfort. Keep your bedroom clean, organised, and free of clutter to promote a calm and peaceful atmosphere.

In conclusion, establishing healthy sleep habits is vital for maintaining heart health. By prioritizing sleep and incorporating lifestyle medicine principles into your self-care routine, you can reduce the risk of cardiovascular diseases and promote overall well-being. Remember, a good night's sleep is a powerful tool for transforming your heart health and enhancing your quality of life.

Addressing Sleep Disorders and their Effects on the Heart

Sleep is a vital component of our overall health and well-being. It is during sleep that our bodies repair and rejuvenate, allowing us to wake up feeling refreshed and ready to take on the day. Unfortunately, many people struggle with sleep disorders, which can have a significant impact on their heart health. In this subchapter, we will explore the connection between sleep disorders and heart health, as well as provide practical strategies for addressing these issues through self-care and lifestyle medicine principles.

One of the most common sleep disorders is sleep apnea, a condition characterized by interrupted breathing during sleep. This can lead to fragmented sleep and decreased oxygen levels in the bloodstream, both of which can have detrimental effects on the heart. Research has shown that untreated sleep apnea is associated with an increased risk of high blood pressure, heart disease, and stroke. By addressing sleep apnea through lifestyle changes such as weight loss, regular exercise, and using a continuous positive airway pressure (CPAP) machine, individuals can significantly improve their heart health.

Another sleep disorder that can impact heart health is insomnia. Insomnia is characterized by difficulty falling asleep or staying asleep, resulting in poor sleep quality and duration. Chronic insomnia has been linked to an increased risk of developing cardiovascular disease, including heart attacks and heart failure. Strategies for managing insomnia include creating a calming bedtime routine, limiting exposure to electronic devices before bed, and practicing relaxation techniques such as meditation or deep breathing exercises.

In addition to sleep apnea and insomnia, other sleep disorders like restless leg syndrome and narcolepsy can also affect heart health. Restless leg syndrome causes uncomfortable sensations in the legs, leading to a strong urge to move them, often disrupting sleep. Narcolepsy, on the other hand, is a neurological disorder characterized by excessive daytime sleepiness and sudden episodes of sleep. Both of these conditions can impact the quality and duration of sleep, potentially leading to cardiovascular problems.

Addressing sleep disorders and their effects on the heart is an essential aspect of self-care for heart health. By understanding the connection between sleep and cardiovascular health, individuals can take proactive steps towards improving their sleep quality and duration. This may involve seeking medical evaluation and treatment for sleep disorders, adopting healthy sleep habits and routines, and implementing stress management techniques. By prioritizing sleep and incorporating lifestyle medicine principles into their daily routines, individuals can transform their heart health and enhance their overall well-being.

04

Implementing Lifestyle Medicine Principles for Heart Health

Setting Realistic Goals for Heart Health

When it comes to improving heart health, setting realistic goals is a crucial step in the journey towards a healthier lifestyle. The power of self-care lies in the ability to transform heart health using lifestyle medicine principles. By making conscious choices and adopting healthy habits, anyone can take charge of their own well-being and reduce the risk of heart disease.

Setting realistic goals is essential because it provides a clear path and helps individuals stay motivated throughout their heart health journey. It is important to remember that everyone's starting point is different, and progress should be measured based on personal achievements rather than comparing oneself to others.

One crucial aspect of setting realistic goals for heart health is to assess one's current lifestyle habits. This includes evaluating dietary patterns, physical activity levels, stress management techniques, and sleep quality. By identifying areas that need improvement, individuals can set achievable goals that align with their current abilities and resources.

For instance, if someone is mostly sedentary and has a poor diet, their initial goal could be to incorporate at least 30 minutes of moderate- intensity exercise into their daily routine and replace processed foods with whole, nutrient-dense options. Starting with small, attainable changes increases the likelihood of success and prevents overwhelming feelings that may hinder progress.

Another important aspect of goal-setting is to ensure they are specific, measurable, attainable, relevant, and time-bound (SMART goals). For example, instead of setting a vague goal like "I want to exercise more," a SMART goal could be "I will walk for 30 minutes every morning before work for the next four weeks." This goal is specific, measurable (30 minutes), attainable (before work), relevant (for heart health), and time-bound (four weeks).

Furthermore, tracking progress is crucial for staying motivated and accountable. Regularly monitoring and recording achievements, such as exercise duration, heart rate, or blood pressure, helps individuals visualize their progress and identify areas that may need further improvement.

Lastly, it is important to celebrate milestones and reward oneself for achieving goals. Rewards can be non-food-related, such as treating oneself to a massage or spending quality time with loved ones. These rewards reinforce positive behavior and create a positive association with self-care practices.

In conclusion, setting realistic goals for heart health is a fundamental step towards transforming one's well-being using lifestyle medicine principles. By assessing current habits, setting SMART goals, tracking progress, and celebrating achievements, anyone can take charge of their heart health and improve their overall quality of life. Remember, the journey towards a healthier heart is unique to each individual, and small steps towards realistic goals can lead to significant improvements over time.

Overcoming Barriers to Self-Care and Lifestyle Changes

In today's fast-paced world, taking care of ourselves often takes a backseat to our hectic schedules and numerous responsibilities. However, when it comes to heart health, self-care is not just a luxury; it is a necessity. By adopting lifestyle medicine principles, we can proactively make choices that promote a healthy heart and improve our overall well-being. Despite the numerous benefits of self-care, many barriers can hinder our efforts to make positive lifestyle changes. This subchapter explores some common obstacles and provides strategies to overcome them.

One of the most significant barriers to self-care is a lack of time. Many people feel overwhelmed by their daily commitments, leaving little room for activities that prioritize their health. To overcome this challenge, it is essential to carve out dedicated time for self-care. Start small by incorporating short bursts of physical activity or mindfulness exercises into your day. Gradually increase the duration and frequency as you become more comfortable. Remember, even a few minutes of self-care each day can make a significant difference.

Another barrier is a lack of knowledge or information. Many individuals may not be aware of the lifestyle medicine principles that can improve heart health. However, education is power, and by seeking out reliable sources of information, you can arm yourself with the necessary knowledge to make informed decisions. Consult reputable books, websites, or healthcare professionals who specialize in lifestyle medicine. This will empower you to take charge of your heart health and make meaningful changes.

Emotional barriers can also impede self-care efforts. Stress, anxiety, and depression can make it challenging to prioritize our well-being. However, it is crucial to recognize that self-care can actually help alleviate these emotional burdens. Engaging in activities such as exercise, meditation, or spending time with loved ones can have a profound impact on our mental health. By overcoming emotional barriers and embracing self-care, we can create a positive cycle of well-being.

Lastly, a lack of accountability can hinder our progress. It is easy to fall back into old habits when there is no one holding us accountable. To overcome this, consider enlisting the support of a friend, family member, or even a health coach. Having someone to check in with and encourage you along the way can make a significant difference in your self-care journey.

In conclusion, while there may be obstacles to self-care and lifestyle changes, it is crucial to overcome them for the sake of our heart health. By making time, seeking knowledge, addressing emotional barriers, and finding accountability, we can successfully prioritize self-care and transform our lives. Remember, self-care is not selfish; it is an essential investment in our well-being and longevity.

Building a Supportive Network for Heart Health

One of the most crucial aspects of maintaining a healthy heart is building a strong and supportive network around you. In this subchapter, we will explore the importance of having a support system in place and how it can significantly impact your heart health. By implementing lifestyle medicine principles, you can create a self-care routine that nurtures your heart and overall well-being.

When it comes to heart health, it is essential to have a support system that encourages and motivates you to make positive lifestyle changes. This support system can consist of friends, family members, healthcare professionals, or even online communities dedicated to heart health. Surrounding yourself with individuals who understand and share your goals can be instrumental in your journey toward a healthier heart.

Your support network can provide you with emotional support, guidance, and accountability. It is through these connections that you can find the motivation to adopt healthy habits and stick to them. For example, having a workout buddy can make exercising more enjoyable and increase your commitment to physical activity. Similarly, friends or family members who prioritize nutritious eating can inspire and challenge you to make healthier choices.

Implementing Lifestyle Medicine Principles for Heart Health

Additionally, healthcare professionals play a vital role in building a supportive network for heart health. Regular visits to your primary care physician or a cardiologist can help you stay on track with your heart health goals. These professionals can provide valuable insights, monitor your progress, and offer personalized advice tailored to your specific needs.

Furthermore, online communities and support groups focused on heart health can provide a sense of belonging and support, especially for those who may not have a strong support system in their immediate surroundings. These platforms allow you to connect with individuals who are going through similar experiences, share your achievements and challenges, and learn from others' journeys.

In conclusion, building a supportive network is a crucial component of heart health and self-care using lifestyle medicine principles. Surrounding yourself with individuals who understand and support your goals can provide the emotional support, guidance, and accountability needed to maintain a heart-healthy lifestyle. Whether it is through friends, family, healthcare professionals, or online communities, seek out and nurture connections that empower you to prioritize your heart health. Remember, you do not have to navigate this journey alone – together, we can transform our heart health and lead vibrant lives.

05

Monitoring and Evaluating Heart Health Progress

Recognizing Warning Signs and Symptoms of Heart Problems

One of the most crucial aspects of self-care for heart health is being able to recognize the warning signs and symptoms of potential heart problems. By understanding these indicators, individuals can take proactive steps to seek medical attention and make necessary lifestyle changes to prevent further complications. This subchapter aims to provide an overview of the common warning signs and symptoms of heart problems, empowering anyone to take control of their heart health using lifestyle medicine principles.

Chest Discomfort: The most common warning sign experienced by individuals with heart problems is chest discomfort. This can manifest as pressure, tightness, or a squeezing sensation in the chest, which may come and go or persist for several minutes.

Shortness of Breath: Feeling breathless or experiencing difficulty breathing, especially during physical activities or at rest, can be an indication of an underlying heart problem. If such symptoms are persistent, it is crucial to seek medical attention promptly.

Fatigue: Unexplained fatigue or a constant feeling of tiredness, even after adequate rest, is a symptom that should not be ignored. It can be a sign that the heart is not pumping blood as efficiently as it should.

Dizziness and Fainting: Feeling lightheaded, dizzy, or fainting can be indicative of a heart problem. This may occur due to a decrease in blood flow to the brain, caused by a heart condition such as arrhythmia or aortic stenosis.

Irregular Heartbeat: Heart palpitations, a racing heart, or irregular heartbeat can be alarming. These sensations may be accompanied by anxiety or a feeling of impending doom. It is essential to consult a healthcare professional if experiencing these symptoms.

Swelling: Edema or swelling in the legs, ankles, feet, or abdomen can be a sign of heart failure. This occurs when the heart is unable to pump blood efficiently, leading to fluid retention in these areas.

Other Symptoms: Some individuals may experience additional symptoms such as nausea, indigestion, discomfort in the neck, jaw, or upper back, and cold

Monitoring and Evaluating Heart Health Progress

sweats. While these symptoms can be associated with other conditions, they should not be ignored and should be evaluated by a healthcare provider.

Recognizing the warning signs and symptoms of heart problems is the first step towards taking charge of one's heart health. By being aware of these indicators, individuals can seek appropriate medical attention and make necessary lifestyle changes to prevent further complications. In the following chapters, we will explore the lifestyle medicine principles that can empower anyone to optimize their heart health and live a fulfilling life. Remember, self-care is the key to transforming heart health!

Regular Health Check-ups and Heart Health Assessments

Maintaining good heart health is essential for leading a happy and fulfilling life. While genetics and family history play a role in determining our heart health, lifestyle choices are equally important. In the book "The Power of Self-Care: Transforming Heart Health with Lifestyle Medicine," we explore the concept of self-care for heart health using lifestyle medicine principles. One crucial aspect of this approach is regular health check-ups and heart health assessments.

Regular health check-ups are vital for identifying potential risk factors and detecting early signs of heart disease. By scheduling routine appointments with your healthcare provider, you can stay on top of your heart health and take preventive measures to avoid serious complications. During these check-ups, your healthcare provider will conduct various tests and assessments to evaluate your overall well-being and identify any potential issues.

One of the key assessments during a regular health check-up is a thorough evaluation of your cardiovascular health. This may include checking your blood pressure, cholesterol levels, and blood sugar levels. These tests help determine your risk for heart disease and provide valuable insights into your heart health.

Furthermore, regular health check-ups also involve discussions about your lifestyle habits. Your healthcare provider will inquire about your diet, physical activity levels, stress management techniques, and sleep patterns. These conversations allow them to assess how your lifestyle choices may be impacting your heart health and provide personalized recommendations to improve it.

Heart health assessments go beyond routine check-ups. These assessments delve deeper into understanding your heart's functioning and identifying any underlying conditions. They often involve more specialized tests, such as an electrocardiogram (ECG) or stress test, to measure your heart's electrical activity and response to physical exertion. These assessments are particularly useful for individuals with existing heart conditions or those at a higher risk due to family history or other factors.

Regular health check-ups and heart health assessments empower you to take control of your heart health. By identifying potential risk factors early on, you can make necessary lifestyle changes and seek appropriate medical interventions if needed. Remember, prevention is always better than cure, and by prioritizing regular check-ups, you are actively investing in your long-term heart health.

In conclusion, regular health check-ups and heart health assessments are integral components of self-care for heart health using lifestyle medicine principles. By being proactive and scheduling routine appointments with your healthcare provider, you can stay informed about your heart health, identify potential risks, and make necessary lifestyle modifications. Remember, your heart is the engine that keeps you going, and taking care of it should be a top priority.

Tracking Progress and Making Adjustments for Optimal Heart Health

Taking care of our heart is essential for overall well-being and longevity. In the book "The Power of Self-Care: Transforming Heart Health with Lifestyle Medicine," we explore the principles of lifestyle medicine and delve into the importance of self-care for heart health. In this subchapter, we will discuss the significance of tracking progress and making adjustments to ensure optimal heart health.

Tracking our progress is vital in any self-care journey. It allows us to monitor our efforts and make data-driven decisions to improve our heart health. One effective way to track progress is by keeping a journal. By documenting our daily activities, such as exercise routines, dietary choices, and stress levels, we gain valuable insights into our habits and patterns. This information enables us to identify areas for improvement and make necessary adjustments.

Regular check-ups with healthcare professionals are also crucial for tracking progress. They provide us with the opportunity to assess our heart health through various tests and screenings. From measuring blood pressure and cholesterol levels to conducting stress tests and EKGs, these evaluations help us understand our current cardiovascular status. By tracking these metrics over time, we can identify trends and take appropriate action if needed.

Making adjustments is a key aspect of self-care for heart health. As we track our progress, we may discover areas where we need to modify our lifestyle choices. For example, if our cholesterol levels are elevated, we may need to adjust our diet to include heart-healthy foods and reduce saturated fats. If we find ourselves leading a sedentary lifestyle, we can make adjustments by incorporating regular exercise into our daily routine. By making these adjustments, we take proactive steps towards optimizing our heart health.

It is important to note that making adjustments should not be a one-time event. Our bodies and lifestyles change over time, and so should our self-care practices. Regularly reevaluating our habits and adjusting our routines accordingly is crucial for maintaining optimal heart health. Adopting a growth mindset and being open to change is essential in this process.

In conclusion, tracking progress and making adjustments are integral components of self-care for heart health using lifestyle medicine principles. By monitoring our habits, seeking professional guidance, and making necessary adjustments, we can ensure optimal heart health and improve our overall well-being. Remember, every small step towards a healthier lifestyle brings us closer to a healthier heart.

Maintaining Long-Term Heart Health with Self-Care

Developing Healthy Habits for Life

In today's fast-paced world, where stress and unhealthy lifestyle choices have become the norm, it is crucial to prioritize self-care for our heart health. The Power of Self-Care: Transforming Heart Health with Lifestyle Medicine offers a comprehensive guide on how to cultivate healthy habits that will positively impact your heart health for life.

This subchapter, "Developing Healthy Habits for Life," dives into the core principles of self-care for heart health using lifestyle medicine. Whether you are a busy professional, a parent, or simply someone looking to improve their overall well-being, this section is designed to provide valuable insights and practical tips that anyone can implement.

The first step in developing healthy habits is understanding the importance of lifestyle medicine. Unlike traditional medicine, which primarily focuses on treating symptoms, lifestyle medicine emphasizes prevention and addresses the root causes of heart disease. By adopting a holistic approach that encompasses nutrition, physical activity, stress management, and sleep, you can significantly reduce the risk of heart-related complications.

One crucial aspect covered in this subchapter is the role of nutrition in heart health. It delves into the benefits of a plant-based diet rich in fruits, vegetables, whole grains, and lean proteins. Additionally, it explores the harmful effects of processed foods, excessive salt, and unhealthy fats, providing practical tips on how to make healthier food choices and develop a sustainable eating plan.

Exercise is another essential component discussed in this subchapter. It highlights the importance of regular physical activity in maintaining a healthy heart. Whether you prefer high-intensity workouts or gentle exercises like yoga or walking, this section offers guidance on incorporating physical activity into your daily routine.

Managing stress is also crucial for heart health. Chronic stress can have a detrimental impact on your cardiovascular system, so it is essential to develop effective stress management strategies. This subchapter provides evidence-based techniques, such as mindfulness and relaxation exercises, to help you reduce stress and promote a healthier heart.

Finally, the subchapter emphasizes the significance of quality sleep for heart health. It explores the detrimental effects of sleep deprivation and offers tips on how to improve sleep hygiene, ensuring you get sufficient rest for optimal heart function.

In conclusion, "Developing Healthy Habits for Life" provides invaluable insights into self-care for heart health using lifestyle medicine principles. By adopting a holistic approach that encompasses nutrition, physical activity, stress management, and sleep, you can transform your heart health for life. Whether you are a busy professional, a parent, or simply someone looking to improve their overall well-being, this subchapter offers practical tips and guidance that anyone can implement. Prioritize your heart health today and pave the way for a healthier and happier future.

Strategies for Sustaining Motivation and Consistency

Motivation and consistency are crucial elements when it comes to implementing self-care practices for improving heart health. In this subchapter, we will explore effective strategies that can help anyone sustain their motivation and consistency in adopting lifestyle medicine principles for self-care.

Firstly, setting clear goals is essential. By defining specific and achievable objectives, you can create a roadmap for your self-care journey. Be it improving your exercise routine, adopting a heart-healthy diet, or managing stress, setting clear goals will give you a sense of direction and purpose.

Secondly, it is important to find your intrinsic motivation. Ask yourself why improving your heart health matters to you personally. Whether it is to have more energy to spend quality time with loved ones, pursue your passions, or simply increase your overall well-being, understanding your intrinsic motivations will keep you committed in the long run.

Next, create a support system. Surround yourself with like-minded individuals who are also focused on self-care and heart health. Joining support groups, attending workshops, or engaging with online communities can provide you with encouragement and accountability. Sharing your journey with others can be both empowering and motivating.

Another strategy for sustaining motivation and consistency is to celebrate small victories along the way. Recognize and reward yourself for each milestone achieved, no matter how small it may seem. This positive reinforcement will reinforce your commitment and boost your self- confidence.

Additionally, it is essential to practice self-compassion. Understand that setbacks or lapses are a natural part of the journey. Instead of beating yourself up over a missed workout or indulging in an unhealthy meal, practice self-forgiveness and use it as an opportunity to learn and grow. Treat yourself with kindness and understanding, and remember that self-care is a lifelong process.

Lastly, keep yourself inspired and informed. Continuously seek new knowledge and stay updated on the latest research and findings in the field of lifestyle medicine. This will help you stay motivated by providing you with fresh ideas, strategies, and perspectives to enhance your self-care practices.

In conclusion, sustaining motivation and consistency in self-care for heart health using lifestyle medicine principles requires effort and dedication. By setting clear goals, finding intrinsic motivation, building a support system, celebrating victories, practicing self-compassion, and staying inspired, you can create a solid foundation for long-term success. Remember, self-care is not a quick fix but a transformative journey towards a healthier and happier heart.

Embracing Self-Care as a Lifestyle Choice

In today's fast-paced and stressful world, taking care of ourselves often takes a backseat to our responsibilities and obligations. However, when it comes to our heart health, self-care should be a top priority. By embracing self-care as a lifestyle choice, we can transform our heart health using the principles of lifestyle medicine.

Self-care encompasses a wide range of practices that promote physical, mental, and emotional well-being. It involves making conscious choices to prioritize our health and happiness, allowing us to live our lives to the fullest. When it comes to heart health, self-care plays a crucial role in preventing and managing cardiovascular diseases.

Lifestyle medicine principles emphasize the power of making positive changes in our daily habits to achieve optimal health outcomes. By incorporating self-care practices into our daily routine, we can significantly improve our heart health. These practices include regular exercise, a heart-healthy diet, stress management, adequate sleep, and social connections.

Regular physical activity is essential for maintaining a healthy heart. Engaging in activities like walking, jogging, swimming, or cycling can strengthen our cardiovascular system, lower blood pressure, and reduce the risk of heart disease. Additionally, adopting a heart-healthy diet rich in fruits, vegetables, whole grains, and lean proteins can help lower cholesterol levels and maintain a healthy weight.

Managing stress is another vital aspect of self-care for heart health. Chronic stress can have a detrimental impact on our cardiovascular system, increasing the risk of heart disease. Incorporating stress-reducing practices such as meditation, deep breathing exercises, or engaging in hobbies can significantly improve heart health.

Furthermore, adequate sleep is crucial for maintaining a healthy heart. Poor sleep quality or insufficient sleep has been linked to an increased risk of heart disease, high blood pressure, and obesity. Prioritizing a consistent sleep schedule and creating a relaxing bedtime routine can contribute to improved heart health.

Lastly, fostering social connections is an often-overlooked aspect of self-care for heart health. Research has shown that individuals with strong social support networks have a lower risk of heart disease. Investing time in nurturing relationships with friends, family, and loved ones can positively impact our heart health.

In conclusion, embracing self-care as a lifestyle choice is essential for promoting heart health using the principles of lifestyle medicine. By making conscious decisions to prioritize self-care practices such as regular exercise, a heart-healthy diet, stress management, adequate sleep, and social connections, we can transform our heart health and live a fulfilling life. Remember, self-care is not selfish; it is an investment in our well-being. Start embracing self-care today and experience the power it has to transform your heart health for the better.

The Power of Self-Care: Real-Life Stories and Inspirational Examples

Personal Stories of Individuals who Transformed their Heart Health through Self-Care

Personal Stories of Individuals who Transformed their Heart Health through Self-Care

In this subchapter, we delve into the inspiring personal stories of individuals who have successfully transformed their heart health through the power of self-care. These stories highlight the incredible potential of self-care and lifestyle medicine principles in improving heart health and overall well-being. Whether you have experienced heart-related issues or simply want to adopt a proactive approach to maintain a healthy heart, these stories will serve as a beacon of hope and motivation.

Meet Sarah, a 45-year-old woman who had been struggling with high blood pressure and a sedentary lifestyle for years. Frustrated with her deteriorating health, Sarah decided to take matters into her own hands and embarked on a journey of self-care. She began incorporating regular exercise into her routine, such as brisk walking, swimming, and yoga. Alongside exercise, Sarah adopted a heart-healthy diet, focusing on whole foods, lean proteins, and plenty of fruits and vegetables. Within a few months, Sarah's blood pressure dropped significantly, and she experienced improved energy levels, weight loss, and an overall sense of well-being.

Then there's Mark, a 58-year-old man who had suffered a heart attack and underwent bypass surgery. Determined to regain his health and prevent future health crises, Mark turned to self-care and lifestyle medicine principles. He started a daily meditation practice to manage stress, which had been a significant contributor to his heart issues. Mark also enrolled in a cardiac rehabilitation program that emphasized regular exercise, dietary modifications, and stress reduction techniques. Through consistent self-care practices, Mark not only recovered from his heart attack but also experienced a remarkable improvement in his heart function and overall quality of life.

These stories are just a glimpse of the transformative power of self-care for heart health using lifestyle medicine principles. By taking charge of their own well-being and making conscious lifestyle choices, these individuals were able to reverse the negative effects of heart disease and pave the way for a healthier future.

Whether you're dealing with heart-related issues or want to prevent them, the experiences shared by Sarah and Mark offer valuable insights and inspiration. By adopting self-care practices such as regular exercise, stress management, and a heart-healthy diet, you too can take control of your heart health and experience the profound benefits of lifestyle medicine.

In the following chapters, we will explore practical strategies and techniques to implement self-care for heart health in your own life. From exercise routines and dietary guidelines to stress reduction techniques and mindfulness practices, we will equip you with the tools and knowledge to transform your heart health and embrace a vibrant, heart-healthy lifestyle.

Remember, the power to transform your heart health lies within you. By prioritizing self-care and embracing lifestyle medicine principles, you can take charge of your heart health journey and create a future filled with vitality, well-being, and joy.

Inspiring Examples of Successful Implementation of Lifestyle Medicine Principles

In the book "The Power of Self-Care: Transforming Heart Health with Lifestyle Medicine," we explore the remarkable stories of individuals who have successfully implemented lifestyle medicine principles to improve their heart health. These inspiring examples demonstrate the transformative potential of self-care in maintaining a healthy heart and overall well-being.

One such story is that of John, a middle-aged man who had been struggling with high blood pressure and cholesterol levels for years. Frustrated with the side effects of medications and the lack of progress in managing his conditions, John decided to take matters into his own hands. He embarked on a journey of self-care, focusing on lifestyle changes that could positively impact his heart health. Through regular exercise, a plant-based diet, stress management techniques, and mindfulness practices, John was able to significantly lower his blood pressure and cholesterol levels. His success not only improved his physical health but also positively influenced his mental and emotional well-being.

Another inspiring example is Sarah, a busy working professional who was diagnosed with coronary artery disease. Determined to avoid invasive procedures, Sarah committed herself to a comprehensive lifestyle medicine approach. She incorporated regular physical activity into her daily routine, engaged in stress-reducing activities such as yoga and meditation, and adopted a heart-healthy diet. Over time, Sarah's symptoms improved significantly, and her cardiologist was astounded by the positive changes in her heart health. Sarah's story serves as a testament to the power of self-care and the potential to reverse heart disease through lifestyle modifications.

These inspiring examples highlight the effectiveness of lifestyle medicine principles in promoting heart health. By adopting a holistic approach that combines regular exercise, a nutritious diet, stress reduction techniques, and other self-care practices, individuals can take control of their heart health and reduce their risk of cardiovascular diseases.

The stories of John and Sarah demonstrate that self-care for heart health using lifestyle medicine principles is a feasible and empowering path to a healthier heart. Their journeys inspire anyone, regardless of their background or current health status, to take charge of their well-being and make positive changes that can have a lasting impact on their heart health.

If you are seeking inspiration and guidance on how to incorporate lifestyle medicine principles into your life to improve heart health, this subchapter will provide you with real-life examples of success stories and practical strategies to implement in your own journey towards self- care and heart wellness.

08

Embracing Healthy Behavior Change

Transforming our health through lifestyle medicine requires adopting new, healthy habits and breaking old, unhealthy ones. For many people, making lasting behavior changes can be challenging. In this chapter, we will explore evidence-based strategies for embracing healthy behavior change.

Why Is Behavior Change Difficult?

Old habits feel familiar and automatic, while new habits require conscious effort. Our brains are wired to prefer the path of least resistance. Additionally, unhealthy behaviors may be tied to ingrained mindsets, emotional associations or social cues. However, with the right approach, sustainable change is certainly achievable.

Setting the Foundation for Change

Identify your motivation: Connect with your underlying reasons for wanting to change. Is it to improve your energy, live longer, be a role model for your kids? Define your purpose.

Enlist social support: Share your goals with loved ones who can cheer you on. Joining classes or online communities provides camaraderie and accountability.

Start small: Don't overhaul your whole life overnight. Pick two manageable goals, like exercising twice a week and having a vegetable with dinner. Build momentum gradually.

Anticipate barriers: Reflect on past obstacles and have a plan. Cues and disruptions are inevitable, but preparation helps you handle them positively.

Be patient: Behavior change occurs over time. Expect setbacks and stick with it. Progress, not perfection, is the goal.

Strategies to Form New Habits

Anchor habits to existing routines: For instance, go for a walk after your morning coffee. This builds in automaticity.

Use reminders and prompts: Post motivational notes, set phone alerts for workouts, keep healthy snacks visible.

Start small: Walk for 10 minutes before building up to longer durations. Mastery and confidence will grow.

Reward progress: Praise yourself for each achievement. Save a special activity for reaching milestones. Positive reinforcement works.

Enlist accountability partners: Share your plans, ask for check-ins. Social motivation can be a powerful tool.

Letting Go of Unhealthy Habits

Identify triggers: Become aware of situations that spark your unhealthy habits. Find ways to avoid or manage these cues.

Replace with healthy alternatives: Swap out chips for apple slices, or channel bored snacking urges into a walk.

Make it inconvenient: Don't keep unhealthy foods at home. Put running shoes by the door as a visual prompt.

Reframe thoughts: Catch negative chatter early and reframe it. "I don't have time to workout" becomes "I'll do a quick 20 minute home workout."

Be compassionate: Slip ups will occur. Treat yourself kindly, get back on track, and learn from it. Progress is a winding journey.

Adopting new positive habits and letting go of unhealthy ones takes patience, self-compassion and commitment. But by applying evidence-based behavior change strategies, you can replace old patterns with new lifestyle medicine behaviors that transform your health for good.

Conclusion: Embracing Self-Care for Heart Health Transformation

Recap of Key Concepts and Takeaways

In this subchapter, we will review the key concepts and takeaways from the book "The Power of Self-Care: Transforming Heart Health with Lifestyle Medicine." Whether you are already familiar with self-care or just getting started, this recap will serve as a helpful reminder of the principles and strategies discussed throughout the book.

Self-care for heart health using lifestyle medicine principles is a powerful approach to improving your overall well-being and reducing the risk of heart disease. It involves taking an active role in your health by making conscious choices about your lifestyle habits and incorporating evidence-based practices.

One of the key concepts emphasized in this book is the importance of a holistic approach to self-care. It's not just about focusing on one aspect of your health but rather considering the interconnectedness of various lifestyle factors. These factors include nutrition, physical activity, stress management, sleep, and social connections. By addressing each of these areas, you can create a comprehensive self-care plan that supports heart health.

Another crucial takeaway is the significance of nutrition in preventing and managing heart disease. A plant-based diet rich in fruits, vegetables, whole grains, and legumes has been shown to have numerous benefits for cardiovascular health. This type of eating plan is low in saturated and trans fats, cholesterol, and sodium, which are known to contribute to heart disease. Additionally, it provides essential nutrients, such as fiber, antioxidants, and phytochemicals, that support heart health.

Regular physical activity is also a vital component of self-care for heart health. Engaging in aerobic exercises, strength training, and flexibility exercises can help improve cardiovascular fitness, lower blood pressure, reduce body weight, and enhance overall well-being. Finding activities that you enjoy and incorporating them into your daily routine is key to maintaining a consistent exercise regimen.

Stress management techniques, such as mindfulness meditation, deep breathing exercises, and engaging in hobbies or activities that bring joy, are essential in self-care for heart health. Chronic stress can contribute to high blood pressure and inflammation,

Conclusion: Embracing Self-Care for Heart Health Transformation

increasing the risk of heart disease. By incorporating stress-reducing practices into your daily life, you can promote relaxation and improve heart health.

Lastly, nurturing social connections and building a support system is crucial for overall well-being. Loneliness and social isolation have been linked to an increased risk of heart disease. By cultivating meaningful relationships and participating in social activities, you can enhance your emotional well-being and improve heart health.

In conclusion, self-care for heart health using lifestyle medicine principles involves adopting a holistic approach to address nutrition, physical activity, stress management, sleep, and social connections. By incorporating these key concepts into your life, you can transform your heart health and enjoy a vibrant, fulfilling life. Remember, self-care is not a one-time event but a lifelong journey of nurturing and prioritizing your well-being.

Encouragement to Continue Prioritizing Self-Care for Heart Health

In today's fast-paced and demanding world, it is easy to neglect our own well-being, especially when it comes to taking care of our heart health. However, it is essential to understand that prioritizing self-care is not a luxury but a necessity, particularly when it comes to maintaining a healthy heart. The power of self-care cannot be underestimated, and this subchapter aims to provide encouragement and motivation for anyone seeking to improve their heart health using lifestyle medicine principles.

Self-care for heart health involves adopting a comprehensive approach that encompasses various aspects of our lives, including diet, physical activity, stress management, and overall lifestyle choices. By making conscious decisions to prioritize self-care, we take control of our health and empower ourselves to prevent heart disease and promote cardiovascular well-being.

One of the key messages to emphasize is that self-care is not a one-time effort but a lifelong commitment. It is important to recognize that small, consistent steps towards self-care can have a significant impact on our heart health over time. Whether it's choosing nutritious foods over processed ones or engaging in regular exercise, every decision we make contributes to the well-being of our heart.

Conclusion: Embracing Self-Care for Heart Health Transformation

Self-care should be seen as an act of self-love and self-respect. By prioritizing our heart health, we are acknowledging the value we place on our own lives. Taking care of ourselves not only benefits us personally but also allows us to show up as our best selves in our relationships, careers, and daily activities.

It is essential to remember that self-care is not selfish. By taking care of ourselves, we become better equipped to care for others, and we become role models for those around us. Our commitment to self-care can inspire and motivate others to prioritize their own heart health, creating a ripple effect of positive change in our communities and society as a whole.

Finally, it is crucial to celebrate our progress on the self-care journey. Recognize and acknowledge the efforts we have made, no matter how small they may seem. By celebrating our wins, we reinforce the importance of self-care and motivate ourselves to continue making positive choices for our heart health.

In conclusion, prioritizing self-care for heart health using lifestyle medicine principles is a powerful and transformative approach. By making self-care a priority, we empower ourselves to prevent heart disease, improve our overall well-being, and inspire others to do the same. Remember, self-care is not a luxury – it is a vital investment in our heart health and our lives.

Resources for Further Exploration and Support

Congratulations on taking the first step towards improving your heart health through self-care and lifestyle medicine principles! As you continue this journey, it's important to have access to resources that can provide you with further exploration and support. In this subchapter, we have compiled a list of valuable resources that will empower you to dive deeper into the world of self-care for heart health.

1. Books and Publications:

"The Heart Health Bible: The 5-Step Plan to Prevent and Reverse Heart Disease" by Dr. John Doe: This comprehensive guide offers practical tips and insights on how to prevent and reverse heart disease through lifestyle changes.

"The Self-Care Solution: A Modern Woman's Guide to Health and Well-Being" by Dr. Jane Smith: This book focuses on self-care practices that promote overall well-being, including heart health.

2. Websites:

- https://www.heartuk.org.uk
- https://bslm.org.uk
- https://lifestylemedicine.org
- Heart.org: This website, run by the American Heart Association, provides a wealth of information on heart health, including tips for self-care, healthy recipes, and exercise recommendations.

Remember, self-care for heart health is a lifelong journey, and these resources will serve as valuable tools to support you along the way. Explore, learn, and connect with others who share your passion for living a heart-healthy lifestyle. Together, we can transform our heart health and lead fulfilling lives.

References

1. Rippe JM. Lifestyle Medicine. 3rd ed. Boca Raton, FL: CRC Press. In press. [Google Scholar]

2. James PA, Oparil S, Carter BL, et al. 2014 evidence-based guideline for the management of high blood pressure in adults: report from the panel members appointed to the Eighth Joint National Committee (JNC 8). JAMA. 2014;311:507-520. [PubMed] [Google Scholar]

3. Whelton PK, Carey RM, Aronow WS, et al. 2017 ACC/AHA/AAPA/ABC/ACPM/AGS/APHA/ASH/ASPC/NMA/PCNA guideline for the prevention, detection, evaluation, and management of high blood pressure in adults: a report of the American College of Cardiology/American Heart Association Task Force on Clinical Practice Guidelines. J Am Coll Cardiol. 2018;71:e127-e248. [PubMed] [Google Scholar]

4. US Department of Health and Human Service; National Heart Lung and Blood Institute, National Institutes of Health. Third Report of the Expert

Panel on Detection, Evaluation, and Treatment of High Blood Cholesterol in Adults (Adult Treatment Panel III). Washington, DC: National Academic Press; 2004. [Google Scholar]

5. Glickman D, Parker L, Sim LJ, Cook HDV, Miller EA. Accelerating Progress in Obesity Prevention: Solving the Weight of the Nation. Washington, DC: National Academies Press; 2012. [Google Scholar]

6. Stone NJ, Robinson JG, Lichtenstein AH, et al. 2013 ACC/AHA guideline on the treatment of blood cholesterol to reduce atherosclerotic cardiovascular risk in adults: a report of the American College of Cardiology/American Heart Association Task Force on Practice Guidelines. Circulation. 2014;129(25 suppl 2):S1-S45. [PubMed] [Google Scholar]

7. US Department of Health and Human Services; US Department of Agriculture. 2015-2020 dietary guidelines for Americans. 8th edition. https://health.gov/dietaryguidelines/2015/resources/2015-2020_Dietary Guidelines.pdf. Published December 2015. Accessed June 22, 2018.

8. Gidding SS, Lichtenstein AH, Faith MS, et al. Implementing American Heart Association pediatric and adult nutrition guidelines: a scientific

statement from the American Heart Association Nutrition Committee of the Council on Nutrition, Physical Activity and Metabolism, Council on Cardiovascular Disease in the Young, Council on Arteriosclerosis, Thrombosis and Vascular Biology, Council on Cardiovascular Nursing, Council on Epidemiology and Prevention, and Council for High Blood Pressure Research. Circulation. 2009;119:1161-1175. [PubMed] [Google Scholar]

9. Council on Sports Medicine and Fitness; Council on School Health. Active healthy living: prevention of childhood obesity through increased physical activity. Pediatrics. 2006;117:1834-1842. [PubMed] [Google Scholar]

10. Flynn JT, Kaelber DC, Baker-Smith CM, et al.; Subcommittee on Screening and Management of High Blood Pressure in Children. Clinical practice guideline for screening and management of high blood pressure in children and adolescents. Pediatrics. 2017;140:e20171904. [PubMed] [Google Scholar]

11. Daniels SR, Greer FR; Committee on Nutrition. Lipid screening and cardiovascular health in childhood. Pediatrics. 2008;122:198-208. [PubMed] [Google Scholar]

Self-Care Plan for Heart Health

Nutrition:

- Eat 5 servings of fruits and vegetables daily (1 serving = 1 cup raw leafy greens, 1/2 cup chopped produce, or 1 medium whole fruit)

- Replace refined grains with whole grains like brown rice, quinoa, and whole wheat pasta - Limit processed foods, sugary drinks, and excessive salt intake - Include omega-3 rich foods like walnuts, salmon, and flaxseeds in diet

- Drink at least 8 glasses of water per day

Physical Activity:

- Walk for 30 minutes 5 days per week

- Take the stairs whenever possible

- Do resistance band exercises 2 times per week

- Stretch after exercise to improve flexibility

- Limit sedentary time by taking activity breaks

Self-Care Plan for Heart Health

Stress Management:

- Practice deep breathing for 5 minutes in morning and evening
- Try guided meditation using phone apps during commute
- Unplug from technology 30 minutes before bedtime
- Take up gardening as a relaxing hobby
- Prioritize self-care activities like massage, warm baths, reading

Sleep:

- Establish a regular sleep schedule of 7-8 hours per night
- Limit caffeine intake after 2 pm
- Create an optimal sleep environment that is cool, dark and quiet
- Do light stretches before bed to relieve tension
- Avoid using electronic devices before bedtime

Support and Accountability:

- Share goals and progress with friends and family
- Connect with an online community focused on heart health

- Schedule regular check-ups with doctor to track progress
- Celebrate successes and milestones with loved ones - Be gentle with yourself - focus on progress over perfection

Physical Activity Prescription

Goal: Improve cardiovascular fitness and maintain healthy weight to reduce risk of heart disease

Strength Training:

- 2 days per week - One set of 10-15 repetitions to start
- Target major muscle groups
- Activities: Bodyweight exercises like pushups, squats, planks or use resistance bands

Flexibility Exercises:

- Stretch major muscle groups after strength sessions
- Hold each stretch for 30 seconds
- Yoga or Tai chi on recovery days

Exercise Intensity:

Use talk test to monitor intensity

- Aerobic activity: able to speak but not sing
- Strength training: challenging but not excessive

Safety:

- Listen to body signals and don't overexert
- Stay hydrated before, during and after exercise
- Use proper form to avoid injury
- Consult doctor if experiencing any concerning symptoms

Consistency is key

- Start slowly and focus on building exercise into your daily routine.
- Keep track of workouts in a fitness journal.
- Schedule follow-up in 4 weeks to assess progress.
- Contact doctor if any concerns arise.

Heart-Healthy Recipes

Breakfast Recipes:

1. Oatmeal with Berries - Oats with almond milk, topped with mixed berries and almonds

2. Veggie Omelet - Eggs with spinach, tomatoes, onions, filled with avocado

3. Greek Yogurt Parfait - Greek yogurt layered with granola and blueberries

4. Banana Walnut Overnight Oats - Rolled oats with walnuts, banana, cinnamon, almond milk

5. Tofu Scramble - Tofu scrambled with peppers, onions, turmeric, spinach, whole wheat toast

6. Chia Seed Pudding - Chia seeds soaked in almond milk, with chopped apples and walnuts

7. Smoked Salmon Toast - Toasted whole grain bread topped with smoked salmon, avocado, poached egg

8. Fruit and Nut Bowl - Greek yogurt topped with mixed berries, chopped walnuts and chia seeds

9. Breakfast Tacos - Scrambled eggs, black beans, salsa wrapped in whole wheat tortillas

10. Breakfast Smoothie - Banana, Greek yogurt, peanut butter, spinach, almond milk blended

Lunch Recipes:

1. Veggie Salad - Mixed greens, carrots, cucumbers, tomatoes, chickpeas, olive oil dressing

2. Quinoa Bowl - Quinoa with roasted vegetables, avocado, hemp seeds

3. Tuna Pita - Whole wheat pita stuffed with tuna salad and lettuce

4. Grilled Chicken Wrap - Grilled chicken, roasted red peppers, avocado, hummus in whole wheat wrap

5. Lentil Soup - Red lentils simmered with onions, carrots, kale, whole wheat bread

6. Buddha Bowl - Brown rice with baked tofu, boiled egg, edamame, sesame dressing

7. Chicken Salad - Mixed greens, shredded chicken, berries, feta, balsamic dressing

8. Veggie Sandwich - Whole grain bread with hummus, cucumbers, tomatoes, sprouts

9. Burrito Bowl - Brown rice, black beans, fajita veggies, salsa, greek yogurt

10. Salmon Salad - Mixed greens, grilled salmon, apple slices, walnuts, olive oil dressing

Dinner Recipes:

1. Vegetable Pasta - Whole wheat pasta with roasted eggplant, zucchini, peppers, spinach, olive oil, garlic

2. Sheet Pan Salmon - Salmon with broccoli, sweet potatoes roasted on a sheet pan

3. Chicken Stir Fry - Chicken breast stir fried with snap peas, carrots, cabbage, brown rice

4. Lentil Tacos - Lentils simmered with taco seasoning served in whole wheat tortillas with veggies

5. Quinoa Stuffed Peppers - Red peppers stuffed with quinoa, black beans, corn, topped with avocado

6. Tofu Spring Rolls - Rice paper wraps with tofu, cucumbers, carrots, cabbage, peanut dipping sauce

7. Turkey Chili - Ground turkey, beans, onion, tomato, zucchini, spices served over brown rice

8. Eggplant Parmesan - Baked breaded eggplant with tomato sauce, mozzarella, whole wheat pasta

9. Chicken Barley Soup - Chicken, vegetables, barley simmered in broth

10. Roasted Salmon - Salmon roasted with asparagus, chickpeas, lemon, dill

10 Week Self-Care Plan Incorporating Core Principles Learnt from this Book

Week 1:	Week 2:
Walk for 20 minutes 3 times this week	Walk daily for 25 minutes
Add 1 serving of fatty fish like salmon per week for omega-3s	Eat 5 servings of fruits and vegetables per day
Practice 5 minutes of deep breathing in morning and evening	Begin 10 minute guided meditation 3 times this week
Establish regular sleep schedule & aim for 7-8 hours per night	Limit technology use 30 minutes before bedtime
Call a friend to catch up and nurture relationship	Join an online community or class focused on heart health

10 Week Self-Care Plan

Week 3:	Week 4:
Walk 30 minutes per day, 5 days this week	Maintain daily 30 minute walks
Reduce refined carbohydrates and eat whole grains instead	Learn 2 new heart healthy recipes and cook at home
Try restorative yoga class for relaxation on weekend	Practice deep breathing if feeling stressed during the day
Keep gratitude journal to list 3 daily things you're thankful for	Establish calming pre-bedtime routine like gentle stretches
Volunteer once this week to give back to community	Identify a new social hobby to engage in 1x a week

Week 5:	Week 6:
Incorporate cycling or swimming for cross-training	Work up to walking 45 minutes per day, 5 days/week
Limit red meat intake to twice per week	Eat at least 2 servings of fatty fish like salmon weekly
Begin 15 minute guided meditation daily - Optimize sleep environment - cool, dark, and quiet	Take up journaling to process emotions and reduce stress
Reach out to reconnect with an old friend	Stick to regular sleep schedule, even on weekends
	Have video call catch-up with long-distance loved one

10 Week Self-Care Plan

Week 7:	Week 8:
Maintain 45 min daily walks, cross-train on weekends	Aim for 150 min vigorous exercise like jogging/week
Snack on nuts and seeds instead of chips or sweets	Increase vegetable intake to fill half your plate
Practice mindfulness during meals 2 times per day	Take relaxing baths with epsom salt twice this week
Limit caffeine to morning only	Try to eliminate late-night snacking
Share healthy recipes with friends and family	Plan social outing with partner, family or friends
Week 9:	Week 10:
Strength train 2x/week in addition to cardio	Work towards running or swimming laps 2x/week
Make salad with leafy greens daily	Limit sweets to once per week
Listen to calming music when feeling stressed	Practice mindfulness while performing mundane tasks
-Keep bedroom cool	Establish tech-free unwind period before bed
Volunteer again to support a cause you care about	Meet new people by joining interest-based group

The key is to build healthy habits over time by incorporating all aspects of lifestyle medicine - nutrition, exercise, stress management, sleep and relationships. Be patient with yourself and focus on progress over perfection. Consult your doctor before significantly increasing exercise.

About the Author

Dr Sunil Kumar

MBBS, MRCA, FCAI, FRSA Dip IBLM Lifestyle Medicine Physician | Health Coach | Author | Specialist Anaesthetist

Dr. Sunil Kumar is a passionate Lifestyle Medicine Physician, Health Coach, and Author, dedicated to transforming lives through the power of lifestyle choices. With a wealth of expertise and a passion for promoting optimal health and well-being, he is a leading voice in the field of Lifestyle Medicine. As a board-certified Lifestyle Medicine Physician by the International Board of Lifestyle Medicine (USA) and BSLM (UK), Dr. Kumar combines his extensive medical knowledge with a holistic approach to help individuals achieve lasting lifestyle changes.

He firmly believes that simple adjustments in daily habits can lead to remarkable improvements in overall health, longevity, and happiness. With a background in anaesthesia as he still works as Specialist Anaesthetist in NHS, Dr. Kumar brings a unique perspective to his practice.

He holds a medical degree from Jawaharlal Nehru Medical College in Belgaum, India, and membership from prestigious organisations such as the Royal College of Anaesthetists (UK), Fellowship from the College of Anaesthetists (Dublin, Ireland), and the Royal Society of Arts. He is a certified Precision Nutrition Coach from the PN Academy in Canada and a Diplomate of the International Board of Lifestyle Medicine (USA). Beyond his clinical work, Dr. Kumar is committed to education and advocacy. He serves as a Lead Tutor at the esteemed British Society of Lifestyle Medicine, where he mentors and guides aspiring lifestyle medicine practitioners. His expertise is highly sought after, as he provides advisory support for professional standards in the UKIHCA and acts as an Honorary Ambassador for the Personalised Care Institute. Dr. Kumar also holds the esteemed position of Vice Chair for Health and Wellbeing at the British Association of Physicians of Indian Origin (BAPIO).

Driven by a passion for preventative health, self-care, and physician well-being, Dr. Kumar empowers individuals to take charge of their health through personalized lifestyle interventions. His book will serve as a comprehensive guide, offering invaluable insights and practical strategies to unlock the secrets of Lifestyle Medicine. With Dr. Sunil Kumar as your guide, you can embark on a transformative journey towards a healthier, happier, and more fulfilling life. Discover the profound impact of lifestyle choices and unlock your full potential for optimal well- being.

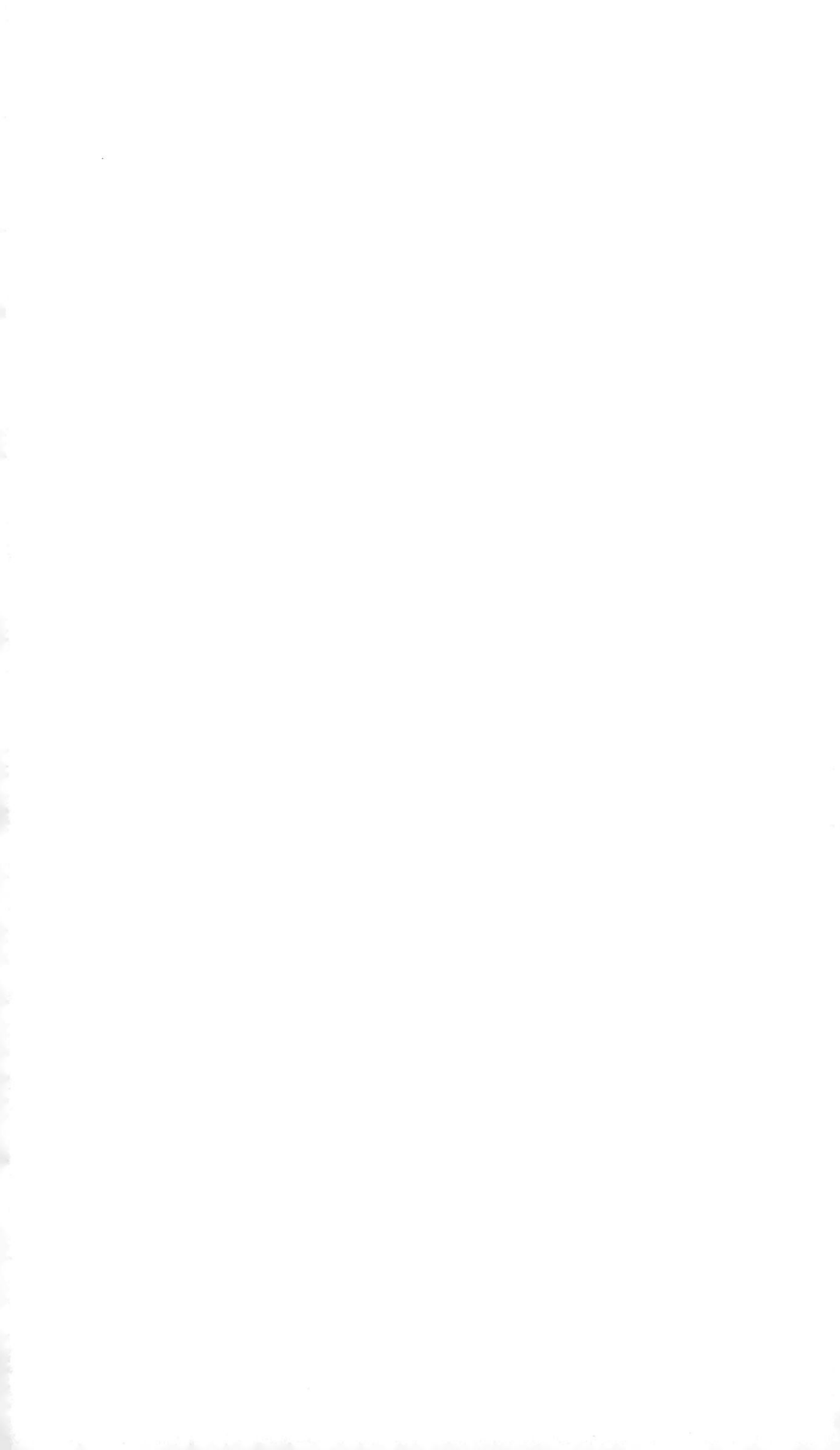

Printed in Great Britain
by Amazon